GROWING

MUSHROOMS

for

PROFIT

Simple and Advanced Techniques for Growing

By William Richards

CONTENTS

MUSHROOMS: PROPERTIES, BENEFITS, CALORIES, USES AND SIDE EFFECTS

Do you know the properties, benefits and uses of mushrooms? For centuries, mushrooms have been known not only as a food but also as a natural remedy. There are also interesting alternative uses of mushrooms in addition to food.

The use of this ingredient in Italian cuisine concerns numerous recipes and in particular the preparation of mushroom risotto, one of the best known and popular dishes based on this food. Many people love mushrooms not only for their flavor but also because they are passionate about their harvesting or cultivation. In fact, some mushrooms can also be grown at home. However, one must never overestimate one's ability to distinguish edible mushrooms from poisonous mushrooms. If in doubt, it is always best to have an expert check the mushrooms you have collected.

Let's discover the properties, benefits, uses and side effects of mushrooms.

MUSHROOMS, PROPERTIES

Mushrooms are a source of carbohydrates, proteins, minerals and vitamins. Among the mineral salts present in mushrooms we find calcium, iron, manganese and selenium. Mushrooms also contain B vitamins and folate.

Among the proteins contained in mushrooms we find lysine and tryptophan. Mushrooms are also a source of antioxidants that are considered useful for the prevention of aging and damage caused to our body by free radicals.

For a long time, it was believed that mushrooms were a food poor in nutrients but scientific studies over the years have noticed that this is not the case and have realized, for example, how much mushrooms are rich in selenium, which is considered important for strengthening the immune system.

In mushrooms we find vitamin B3 which is needed by our body to contribute to the proper functioning of the nervous system and to proper oxygenation of the blood. Vitamin B2 is essential for the production of red blood cells and for metabolism.

Let's summarize the properties of mushrooms:

- ✓ They are a source of mineral salts
- ✓ They contain B vitamins
- ✓ They are a source of vegetable protein
- ✓ They contain carbohydrates
- ✓ They are a source of lysine and tryptophan
- ✓ They bring antioxidants

MUSHROOMS, CALORIES

The caloric intake of mushrooms is not high. For all varieties of mushrooms, it is around 25 kcal per 100 grams of fresh product. Fresh mushrooms can contain water up to 90% of their weight.

MUSHROOMS, NUTRITIONAL VALUES

Mushrooms are primarily a source of protein and carbohydrates. Here is an example of the protein and carbohydrate content for some varieties of mushrooms.

The values of proteins and carbohydrates contained in mushrooms can vary, but we take into account that 100 grams of fresh mushrooms contain about 4 grams of carbohydrates and 2-3 grams of protein.

By way of example, here is the nutritional values per 100 grams of **porcini mushrooms**.

- ✓ Fat g 0.1
- ✓ Carbohydrates g 4.3
- ✓ Protein g 2.5
- ✓ Fibers g 0.6
- ✓ Sugars g 1.72
- ✓ Water g 92.12
- ✓ Ash g 0.98
- ✓ Calcium 18 mg
- ✓ Sodium 6 mg
- ✓ Phosphorus 120 mg
- ✓ Potassium 448 mg
- ✓ Iron 0.4 mg
- ✓ Magnesium mg 9
- ✓ Zinc 1.1 mg

✓ Copper 0.5 mg
✓ Manganese 0.142 mg
✓ Selenium mcg 26

MUSHROOMS, BENEFITS

Mushrooms have always been considered useful for strengthening the immune system, they are used as a natural antibiotic and to protect the body from seasonal ailments.

Some benefits of mushrooms may also relate to the ability to lower bad LDL cholesterol and keep blood cholesterol levels at bay. The intake of mushrooms is considered useful by unconventional medicine especially during the change of seasons to strengthen the body's defences.

Among the main benefits attributed to mushrooms we find their ability to counteract and prevent aging due to their antioxidant content, the ability to prevent cardiovascular disease and to stem the accumulation of cholesterol in the arteries.

Mushrooms can therefore be useful to:

✓ Lower and control cholesterol
✓ Prevent and fight aging
✓ Promote metabolism
✓ Enrich the diet with antioxidants
✓ Prevent cardio-circulatory diseases
✓ Strengthen the immune system
✓ Prevent the accumulation of cholesterol in the arteries

MUSHROOMS RECIPES

Mushrooms are used in the kitchen for the preparation of numerous recipes starting with the famous mushroom risotto. Mushrooms are both an ingredient to season first courses and to enrich second courses and side dishes.

HERE ARE SOME IDEAS AND RECIPES TO PREPARE WITH MUSHROOMS.

- Mushroom risotto
- Pumpkin mushroom and hazelnut sauce
- Recipes with chanterelles
- Lasagne With Mushrooms
- Pasta with mushrooms
- Seitan with mushrooms
- Tofu with mushrooms
- Polenta with mushrooms
- Mushroom cream
- Velvety Mushroom
- Spreadable mushroom sauce
- Mushrooms in Oil
- Salted mushrooms in a pan
- Rice noodles with mushrooms and bamboo
- Rice dumplings with mushrooms
- Potato gnocchi with mushrooms
- Side dish with mushrooms and bamboo

- Baked potatoes with mushrooms
- Cream of mushroom and potatoes
- Rice salad with mushrooms
- Porcini mushroom pizza
- Risotto with mushrooms and pumpkin

MEDICINAL MUSHROOMS

Mushrooms are not just considered an ingredient to be used in cooking. In fact, we talk more and more often about medicinal mushrooms. We will have to wait to understand if in the opinion of science, mushrooms can really be considered 'miraculous'. At the moment we are talking about the prevention of functional imbalances of the organism and of fungi as adjuvants for our physiological functions.

Reishi, or Ganoderma lucidum, also known as the mushroom of immortality is currently one of the varieties that is attracting the most attention from the scientific and natural healing world.

The medicinal mushroom Reishi is antioxidant, anti-inflammatory, antibacterial and antiviral, reduces stress, anxiety and feelings of tiredness, protects the liver, regulates cholesterol, blood sugar and blood pressure and decreases the body's reaction to allergies. This last characteristic is due to the fact that in this mushroom there are ganoderic acids (triterpenes) which limit the production of histamine.

HOW TO GROW MUSHROOMS AT HOME

Did you know that mushrooms can be grown at home? Some Italian schools have already started projects to cultivate mushrooms thanks to the recovery of coffee grounds and now there are real kits for sale, especially in gardening shops and agricultural consortia, and everything needed to grow mushrooms in home and garden.

Mushrooms, alternative uses

Among the alternative uses of mushrooms we find the production of vegetable leather and vegetable fabrics for the production of clothes and accessories. With particular techniques the mushrooms are cultivated and used in order to create a resistant fabric suitable for the manufacture of workable materials that can be used to make clothes and accessories.

Mushrooms, contraindications and side effects

As for the consumption of mushrooms, attention must be paid to allergies, risk of intoxication, risk of consuming poisonous mushrooms, excess in quantities. It all obviously depends on personal tolerance to mushrooms and the ability to recognize edible mushrooms.

It is always essential, in case of doubt, to submit the collected mushrooms to an expert to verify that they cannot cause health risks and that inedible mushrooms have not been collected by mistake.

The yogic diet advises against the consumption of mushrooms because they are considered a food too heavy in terms of energy for both the body and the mind. According to the yogic tradition, those who consume mushrooms may have difficulty concentrating during meditation and negative effects on body and mind.

Anyone who has doubts about the intake of mushrooms and the interaction with the medications they are taking in this period should consult their doctor to understand if some combinations between medicines and mushroom consumption can cause problems.

Reishi mushrooms - Ganoderma lucidum, for example, are not recommended for those who have undergone transplants, for those who take immunosuppressive or anticoagulant and antiplatelet drugs (with particular reference to the Ganoderma lucidum fungus) and for those suffering from allergy to fungi.

Fungi are a large group of living organisms. There are more than 100 thousand species but only a few are edible (good to eat), others are toxic or poisonous. There are also single cell fungi such as yeasts and molds.

UPPER MUSHROOMS AND LOWER MUSHROOMS

Fungi can be microscopic and macroscopic.

Macromycetes mushrooms

The macroscopic ones are also called macromycetes or higher fungi. It is precisely the mushrooms that we commonly known, i.e. those that have such dimensions that they can be observed with the naked eye. Macromycetes Mushrooms are the classic mushrooms that we see and collect.

Micromycetes mushrooms

Microscopic fungi, on the other hand, also called micromycetes or lower fungi, are for example the common molds that attack food or the fungi responsible for antibiotics or fermentations (for example yeast).

Micromycetes mushrooms are "Penicillium" microscopic fungi. Usually, we speak of mushrooms referring to the category of macromycetes and higher fungi. In fact, these are the mushrooms that are collected and cooked.

The world of mushrooms

Fungi include over 100,000 species of organisms that deserve to be categorized into a group of their own. Scholars have decided to form a separate kingdom, that of mushrooms, because these living organisms have particular characteristics.

Some of these characteristics are common to plants, other characteristics are common to the world of animals. However, mushrooms are neither animal nor vegetable. They are organisms halfway between the two groups because they have characteristics of both one and the other group.

Similarities with Plants

Fungi differ from plants because they have no photosynthetic pigments and therefore cannot use the carbon dioxide present in the atmosphere to produce sugar (glucose) as plants do. However, as plants are planted on the ground, they have a similar shape and reproduce with seeds (the spores). They are therefore unable to produce food on their own through photosynthesis, like plants.

Similarities with Animals

With animals, the fungus shares the fact that in order to survive it is forced to consume simple substances produced by others, such as proteins and sugars (such as using decaying dead leaves). Another characteristic that fungi have in common with the animal kingdom is that the fungal cell walls are also formed by chitin which also makes up the exoskeletons of insects.

One last thing:

In short, a fungus can live even without sunlight depending only on other organisms, unlike plants. Here is the difference between autotrophic organisms such as plants and heterotrophic organisms which include animals.

REPRODUCTION OF MUSHROOMS

Now let's talk about the reproduction system that mushrooms have developed and refined over millions of years.

THE HYPHAE AND THE MYCELIUM

What we call fungi are nothing more than a set of microscopic filaments called hyphae. These filaments, the hyphae, intertwine with each other and form the mycelium. Spreading in the soil, the hyphae form a kind of reticular structure that finds fertile ground for development in the woods, in the soil and around the roots of trees.

hyphae of fungi

Development of hyphae in the soil. The mycelium is the vegetative organ of the fungus and provides for the absorption, assimilation and respiration of the fungus.

THE CARPOPHORE BODY

When the mycelium develops and reaches maturity it can give rise to a carpophore body. It is precisely the carpophore, that is the fruiting body of the mushroom, that we see coming out of the ground.

[16]

Therefore, the mycelium of the fungus will give rise to a body of a carpophore only when it reaches maturity and only if the environment and conditions are favorable for its development.

So, it is important to understand that the fungus that we see coming out of the ground is only a fruiting of the mycelium that is actually inside the ground. The purpose of the part that emerges from the ground, the carpophore, is to multiply the species by spreading the spores of the fungus.

This is just one of the reproduction mechanisms that every mushroom has.

Another possibility is that the fungus spreads due to fragmentation of part of the original mycelium. However, the most common means of spreading the spores is that of the wind which can carry them, being very light, even hundreds of kilometers.

Insects also play their part in the distribution of spores, both those parasites of the fungus and insects that occasionally pass through. In this sense, even rabbits and wild boars that eat mushrooms can then shed the indigestible spores along with the excrement.

THE SPORES OF THE FUNGUS

The spores of the fungus are contained within the carpophore. The spores are none other than the seeds of the fungus. Periodically they are released and are carried by wind, water or even by insects or other animals.

PRIMARY AND SECONDARY MYCELIUM

If the spores find optimal soil and conditions, they germinate creating the primary mycelium again. This primary mycelium, if it does not quickly find a primary mycelium of the opposite sex, dies. From this union a compact and new interweaving of hyphae is generated which creates the secondary mycelium and which will therefore lead to the completion of the mushroom reproduction cycle, with the birth of a new carpophore. Fungi can also reproduce asexually through the formation of particular conid cells from which the new secondary mycelia develop directly.

ASCOMYCETES AND BASIDIOMYCETES FUNGI

A fundamental distinction in the realm of higher fungi is that between ascomycete and basidiomycete fungi. It should be known that in higher fungi there are fertile hyphae. The fertile hyphae are found in a specific part of the fruiting body of the fungus and are the ones that can produce the spores.

HYMENIUM

This intertwining of fertile hyphae is called the hymenium. Let's take two examples: in a Porcini Mushroom, which is a mushroom with a tubular fruiting body, the hymenium are the inner surfaces of the tubules. In an Amanita Caesaria mushroom the outer faces of the individual lamellae are the hymenium; the rest of the mushroom is formed by sterile hyphae. The hymenium of boletus is white when young and then turns greenish.

ASCUS AND BASIDIA

At this point the spores are produced by two types of cells, the ascus or the basidia. It is therefore a division based on the different anatomical structures that form the spores. In ascomycetal fungi these spores are produced in a disordered way in the aschi, cylindrical cells that once mature open and allow the spores to disperse.

In basidiomycetes fungi, on the other hand, the hymenium is made up of lamellae or tubes that generally open outwards through small pores. The structures are cylindrical in shape, made from small tubules such as in boletes and spores are formed at their ends.

The shape and color of the spores also have a great variety and are used to determine the species of the fungus. Truffles are part of the ascus class. The basidia, on the other hand, include amanite, russole, porcini mushrooms, etc.

THE 3 MAIN CATEGORIES

Due to the different way they feed and way of life, mushrooms are divided, classified and grouped into three main sub-categories:

Parasitic Mushrooms

Parasitic fungi are organisms that feed on other living organisms. They can feed on trees or shrubs that are already sick or debilitated for the purpose of using their organic material.

Even lower fungi can also develop directly above animals, as do molds. Some species of fungi such as Armillaria mellea can live both saprophytic and parasitic.

Flammulina velutipes velvety agaric

Flammulina Velutipe is both a saprophytic and parasitic fungus. Parasitism between fungus and fungus is widespread among the lower fungi. It is called mycoparasitism and an example is the boletus parasiticus that grows on the Scleroderma aurantium or the Niyctalis asterospora that grows on the fungi of the genus russula. The organisms attacked by parasitic fungi are damaged over time and are no longer able to develop and grow in the best way.

Saprophytic mushrooms

Saprophytic fungi are organisms that feed on waste materials from other living beings or on dead organic materials. *For example:*

Those that grow on top of animal droppings and manure are saprophytic fungi and are called coprophilic and urophilic fungi.

Fungi that grow on wood coals or burnt material are called cinericoli.

Those that live on dead leaves fallen on the ground or on the bark or pine cones fallen to the ground, are always saprophytic fungi.

The species that grow on dead animals are called necrophils. The fungi that grow on humus are saprophytic soil fungi.

Saprophytic fungi can be considered the "scavengers of the forest" because they feed on dead organic material or the waste products of other living organisms.

They are very important because they are able to transform dead organic matter (dry leaves, broken branches, dead animals, excrements) into mineral salts essential for the life of plants.

Symbiotic mushrooms

Finally, there are the symbiotic fungi which are organisms that develop interactions with other organisms in the same environment. The most classic expression of this type of fungi is mycorrhiza, that is the symbiosis between a fungus and a specific plant, tree or bush.

The Mycorrhiza

In this way of living, the fungus attaches itself to the roots of the plant. The situation benefits both organisms because between the two there is an exchange of substances useful for both.

The plant yields to the fungus some organic substances that it is unable to build on its own because it cannot use photosynthesis. For example, carbohydrates or glucose.

The plant, on the other hand, thanks to the union with the fungus and its mycelium, considerably increases the absorbent surface of its roots and therefore receives more water, mineral salts and compounds. It will also benefit from better defences against pests and diseases.

[22]

A type of symbiotic mushroom is the porcini   which can live in symbiosis with numerous broad-leaved trees (chestnut, oak, beech, etc.) and conifers such as fir trees. But mushrooms do not become symbionts only with trees: for example, lichens interact with algae.

Morphology of Mushrooms

How a mushroom is made

The body of the fungi is made up of a set of microscopic filaments called "hypha" which intertwine to form the mycelium.

The hyphae spread through the soil and form a kind of network. From this network the mycelium develops and gives rise to a fruiting body that contains a very large number of spores.

The spores are carried by the wind or by insects or even by water and will give rise to another interweaving of hypha.

MUSHROOMS ANATOMY

Fungi are very particular organisms; they are not classifiable as either plants or animals. Some of the existing species of fungi are microscopic, while others are macroscopic (ie they can be seen as a single organism with the naked eye) and can be collected from the ground. Among these, some can also be eaten, while others are toxic or even poisonous for the human species, being among the most harmful foods of all.

The discussion will focus on the so-called macromycetes, that is the mushrooms that can be seen with the naked eye and are collected, epigeal, that is, which have a well-developed part that comes out of the ground (unlike the hypogeal mushrooms that live all their life underground) and which can therefore be harvested or cultivated.

What is a mushroom

Fungi is the term that refers to a kingdom of the living, the highest classification for living organisms. There are only five kingdoms in nature: bacteria, protists, plants, fungi and animals. The fact that fungi and plants (which are traditionally considered similar) belong to different kingdoms while mosquito and elephant (which are not exactly similar) belong to the same kingdom gives a first idea of the distance between the group of organisms referred to as fungi and all the others.

In fact, fungi have intermediate characteristics between animals and plants: they are distinguished from plants by not being able to create organic compounds by exploiting sunlight, therefore they are not able to carry out chlorophyll photosynthesis; they therefore feed on other organic substances, just like animals. But they also have aspects similar to those of plants, such as the "roots" planted in the ground and the inability to move.

What distinguishes the fungus from other living organisms are the following three characteristics;

• They are heterotrophic ie they cannot synthesize organic compounds by themselves;

• They have no fabric, unlike plants and animals. They have no channels, vessels, transport structures for nutrients; they are just a "mountain" of cells all the same that take on a certain shape as a whole;

• They reproduce through particular structures called spores, therefore without going through an embryonic phase unlike animals (with the embryo) and plants (with the seed). The spores, by sexual reproduction (recombination of two fungi) or asexual (cloning of a single fungus) simply begin to multiply and thus give rise to the new fungus.

Among the many characteristics that distinguish mushrooms, there is also the number of cells that compose them; there are unicellular fungi (such as Saccharomyces cerevisiae, better known as brewer's yeast) and multicellular fungi, based on how many cells they make up; what are traditionally called "fungi" are multicellular organisms.

Fungi can also be distinguished on the basis of their mode of nutrition: parasites, saprophytes or symbionts.

• Parasitic fungi are fungi that live at the expense of other organisms. Generally, they are microscopic fungi (think of those that cause nail fungus, for example) and feed on the substances of other organisms until they kill them. Few of the edible mushrooms do this.

• Saprophytic fungi are fungi that feed on dead organic matter, such as old tree trunks or protein from dead animals on the ground. They are very important fungi for the ecosystem, because their enzymes are able to digest even very hard substances, such as the chitin that forms the exoskeleton of insects; digesting it and then dying make it available to other organisms, such as plants, concluding the cycle of the food chain. Some of the edible mushrooms are saprophytes, such as the famous Champignons (Agaricus bisporus).

• Symbiotic fungi are fungi that live in symbiosis with other organisms, usually with plants. It is a relationship similar to the parasitic one with the difference that both species benefit. Usually, fungi are born on the roots of the plants that host them, and take energy from the plant but at the same time collect substances (usually mineral salts) from the soil and transmit them to the plant, which uses them. They also protect it from attack by parasitic fungi and bacteria. The symbiotic relationship between fungus and plant is called mycorrhiza, and explains why some mushrooms (such as porcini, Boletus edulis) grow only in the presence of specific plants, generally in the woods composed mostly of those plants.

The fungal anatomy

One of the most important characteristics of mushrooms is their shape. Fungi can take different forms, from the well-known "mushroom" shape, therefore stem and cap, to the strangest shapes and this because there are no internal structures, therefore the anatomical parts may be missing or greatly modified in a species, compared to the others.

In fact, in the logic of fungal life, the epigeal part, that is the one that emerges, has the sole reproductive purpose, that of spreading the spores in the surrounding environment and colonizing it.

In any case, most mushrooms exhibit the following structures:

• The cap, the upper part which is important to distinguish the color of the mushroom, the possible presence of parasites and the age;

• The hymenophore, which is the part that is between the gills or in the pores, under the cap, and is the organ where the real spores (hymenium) develop which, falling, will be carried by the wind into the environment;

• Lamellae, pores and quills are the shapes that the part underneath the cap can take and are very important for the recognition of the single fungal species;

• The stem is an elongated part that separates the cap of the mushroom from the ground, to bring up the hymenophore that will spread the spores;

• The volva and the ring are two structures that protect the hymenium in the early stages of growth of the fungus. The volva is located at the base of the stem, and is useful in the early stages of life while the ring, if present, is useful in the more advanced stages, during growth.

Considering the presence, absence, shape, color, consistency of every single part of the mushroom structure, the different species can be distinguished; it is a very important thing to do if you are a collector, but it is also the technique used by ASL mycologists: recognition with molecular methods is still too slow, in particular in cases of poisoning.

Collection and cultivation of mushrooms

Unlike the main known plant and animal species, which are bred or cultivated, two different types of supply are used for mushrooms, due to their particular characteristics: cultivation and harvesting.

Harvesting is the main activity at an amateur level. Even in the trade, however, harvested mushrooms are used: this depends on the fact that some mushrooms simply cannot be grown or it would not be economically advantageous to do so. Porcini mushrooms, for example, being symbiont mushrooms, grow in the vicinity of some very specific species of trees, and their environment cannot be recreated under controlled conditions, which is why porcini are generally collected, and this activity must be subject to very precise laws.

The alternative, valid only for some species of mushrooms, is cultivation: this practice is carried out mainly with saprophytic mushrooms, and the most widespread cultivation is that of champignons. Orecchiette (Pleurotus ostreatus) are also quite common.

Some species of mushrooms can also be grown at home, under controlled conditions, to have edible mushrooms within a few weeks of "sowing".

In any case, cultivation always requires the right substrate, i.e. a soil that contains the nutrients suitable for the fungus to be cultivated (you can do it yourself or buy ready-made soil) and the mycelium, the spores of the fungus, which they buy in small bags in agricultural shops and spread on the substrate waiting for the growth of mushrooms.

Mushrooms: nutritional characteristics

Mushrooms are some of the least nutritious foods of all, due to the substances they contain. They are composed of a lot of water, while the macronutrients are few and their digestion is made difficult by the presence of chitin in the cell wall, a very difficult polysaccharide to digest (it is the same that makes up the exoskeleton, that is the hard shell, of insects).

However, the proteins contained in mushrooms are of good nutritional quality, comparable to those of meat (even if they are very few, three or five grams of protein can be obtained from 100 grams of mushrooms).

Mushrooms are rich in trace elements absorbed by the soil and vitamins that are able to synthesize or absorb by plants.

The main component are proteins, which are of good quality although difficult to extract; even the lipids are of good quality, being mainly represented by so-called essential fatty acids such as linoleic acid, but they are nevertheless so poorly represented (150 grams of mushrooms are equivalent in terms of fat to a gram of oil, one fifth of a teaspoon of tea) which is unlikely to have a preponderant action on the body. On the other hand, the supply of fiber is good, which regulates intestinal transit.

Also interesting are the many trace elements and vitamins that the national institute has not quantified, but which we know are very abundant in mushrooms: among these selenium, sodium, potassium, calcium, iron and manganese as well as vitamins A, D, C, K and some B vitamins, which take part in the various metabolic processes of our body.

Conservation of mushrooms

Since it is not always possible to eat fresh mushrooms (especially those coming from harvesting, which is done only in certain seasons) it is useful to know which conservation methods keep the nutrients better.

• Drying: very common for porcini, it is a method that consists of evaporating the water present in the mushroom. In this way the nutrients remain, but the mushrooms must then be rehydrated in order to be consumed; alternatively, they are used to flavor dishes, crumbled.

• Preservation in oil: this is the most-used technique in the home. It consists of boiling the mushrooms in equal parts of oil and vinegar for a few minutes, then putting them in the jars covered with the cooking liquid. The method disperses many of the nutrients into the liquid itself and can also be dangerous for the eventual development of clostridium botulinum. Absolutely do not consume if you notice the presence of air bubbles in the preserves.

• Freezing: Another very common preservation method is to put the mushrooms in the freezer after washing them to remove the earth. To prevent them from falling apart, it is advisable to store them in the lowest shelf of the freezer, and it is important to cook them still frozen to avoid losing nutrients with defrosting. This is why it is important to wash them before putting them in the freezer.

Main species of mushrooms

In Italy, and even more so, globally, there are many different species of mushrooms. Some are known and sought after, others are little known because they are found only in some areas, or altitudes, and not in others.

PORCINO

Belonging to the genus Boletus, and to the Boletus edulis species, the porcini is a mushroom with excellent edibility compared to others, it has a very intense flavor and goes well with many culinary preparations, in particular those based on meat. It is consumed both fresh and preserved and dried porcini mushrooms are particularly popular. It has a rather high cost compared to that of other mushrooms because it cannot be cultivated as it is not a saprophytic mushroom but a symbiont of the oak and chestnut in the flat areas, beech and fir in the mountain ones. It also develops in groups, if the ideal microclimate is present.

Its edibility is excellent and does not have any kind of contraindication except that, in the harvest phase, it can be confused with other mushrooms. If confused with other species of the genus Boletus, the consequences are generally not serious, except for Boletus satanas: however, this mushroom is of a different color (white cap and red stem, and not a brown cap and yellow stem like the porcini).

It being understood that before consumption it is important to subject it to mycological analysis, a good method of discrimination (which applies only to porcini) can be to cut a small part of it: it must not change color after a few seconds, otherwise we could be in the presence of another species.

CHAMPIGNON

The most widespread mushroom for trade and therefore for consumption is certainly the Champignon, also called French Prataiolo, belonging to the Agaricus bisporus species.

It is a fungus that commonly grows also in Italy, difficult to confuse with other fungal species. It usually grows in meadows, where the fine earth and the presence of small dead plants and insects make it perfect as a habitat: it is in fact a saprophytic fungus. Generally, it is gregarious, that is, you never find a single specimen but a group.

Its second name depends on the fact that the first industrial crops were found in the surroundings of Paris: today it is grown everywhere and throughout the year at a controlled temperature, so much so that it represents up to 80% of all mushrooms cultivated in the world, so it is easy to find in food outlets. The price is also very affordable and this is because its cultivation, unlike other cultivated mushrooms, is advantageous for those who carry it out, allowing prices to be kept at low levels.

The champignon does not have a too intense flavor and its consumption, whether cooked or raw, does not involve dangers; however, for children or pregnant women, it is advisable to eat it cooked to avoid even those rare symptoms that can result from consumption.

OYSTER, MUMPS, CHILBLAINS

Different names for a single mushroom, the Pleurotus ostreatus. It is also a saprophytic mushroom, like Champignon, and also cultivable: it is the second most cultivated mushroom, but the quantities are much lower than the first, about a quarter. It is a fungus that prefers to grow on wood, so it can be found on old stumps of dead trees (where the mycelium develops right on the trunk, with groupings similar to those of oysters, which is why one of its many names it is "Oyster mushroom") and sometimes grows directly in the lower parts of the broad-leaved trees, behaving in any case as a saprophyte on the parts of the bark which are now dead and no longer sprayed by the sap. On the market it is quite commonly found, mainly preserved in oil or frozen, forms in which, moreover, it can be part of the various "mixed mushrooms" that can be found in supermarkets. It has a concave cap, the color of which can vary, well evident gills and a diameter that can range from 5 to 25 centimeters. It is quite common throughout Italy.

Some studies have reported that this mushroom may contain some compounds that have anti-inflammatory or cholesterol-lowering activity, which could indicate the presence of additional beneficial properties.

COCKEREL, CHANTERELLE OR FINFERLO

The Cockerel, with its array of regional names, is one of the most common edible mushrooms in our country and belongs to the Cantharellus cibarius species. However, it is not commonly found on the market because, being a mycozzyric mushroom, therefore a symbiote, it is not possible to cultivate it at advantageous prices for its sale, which is why the only way to find it is to collect it: it is still very common and it can be found in deciduous and coniferous forests at various altitudes. Much appreciated, it has a strong flavor and is used alone or as a side dish. It is inadvisable to eat it raw not so much for the toxic effects (which it does not have, even if the usual recommendations regarding children apply) as because the flavor does not come out except with the effect of cooking which breaks down its cellular structures. It is not dangerous, but the appearance is confused with that of the Omphalotus olearius mushroom, which although it is much larger has a color similar to that of the cockerel and also an appearance that vaguely resembles it. The discriminant is the hymenium, structured in lamellae in the Omphalotus, in crests in the cockerel, but an inexperienced collector can get confused. Omphalotus is poisonous, has short-term symptoms but can also be fatal if consumed in large quantities, which is why it is a good idea to always have them checked by the ASL mycological inspector before consuming the cockerels.

GOOD EGG

Amanita caesarea, the good egg, is one of the mushrooms considered to be the best. Like the other species that cannot be cultivated, it is a symbiotic mushroom, which is found in symbiosis with trees such as chestnut and oak, as long as it is in a dry and mild climate. This is why it is found mainly in Southern Italy and rarely above a thousand meters above sea level. It must be harvested and is highly sought after in the kitchen, where it is eaten both cooked and raw, as a salad. However, it is a fungus in some respects dangerous, mainly due to the possibility of confusing it with other fungi: when it is adult and has a well-opened cap, the intense orange color makes it difficult to confuse it, but in the state of ovum, i.e. when it has emerged from the ground a few days before, it can be confused with other mushrooms belonging to the same species such as Amanita aureola or Amanita muscaria or Amanita phalloides.

The good egg is becoming increasingly rare: despite the law explicitly prohibits the collection of Amanite in the state of ovum, many gatherers do it (also thanks to few forest controls) preventing the fungus from growing and spreading spores in the environment to favor the birth of other specimens.

MUSHROOMS: BENEFICIAL PROPERTIES AND TIPS FOR SAFE CONSUMPTION

Fungi are organisms that are distinct from plants in terms of morphology, vegetative life, properties and reproduction, in fact constituting a kingdom in their own right. However, both because they have different nutritional aspects in common with vegetables, and for their use in the common diet, they are often considered foods of plant origin. They can grow almost anywhere, from woods to meadows, from desert to rocky terrain and even in land burned by fires. The species of mushrooms are innumerable, many poisonous, others edible and with therapeutic properties, each having its own scientific name. The best known from a food point of view are certainly the porcini, the cardoncello, the champignon, the chanterelle and the chiodino, to name a few, each with its own characteristics and unmistakable taste.

Let's find out, then, with the help of Dr. Francesca Evangelisti - nutrition biologist - the properties of mushrooms and what to pay attention to when we decide to consume them.

CALORIES OF MUSHROOMS AND COMPOSITION

"The macronutrient composition, very similar to that of vegetables, is not high", specifies the nutritionist. The most abundant are proteins and carbohydrates, present (although the quantity varies from species to species) in any case in very small quantities (about 4 grams of carbohydrates and 2-3 grams of protein in 100 grams of fresh food). However, "proteins are considered to be of good quality, as are lipids, being mostly represented by essential fatty acids such as linoleic acid". Mushrooms are very rich in water, especially the champignon and ovum varieties (up to 90% of their weight). The fiber content is also good, but it varies according to the species; the black truffle is certainly the richest. The mineral content is not particularly high, except for potassium (especially mushrooms and black truffles) but also iron, selenium, phosphorus, zinc, manganese, calcium, however, the doctor specifies that "a lot depends on the type of soil where the mushrooms they grow ".

On the other hand, the vitamin content is overall good: in particular, in mushrooms we find B12, absent in foods of plant origin, while vitamin A is abundant in chanterelles. There are numerous antioxidants, while the calories of mushrooms are not high: "most species contain about 25 calories per 100 grams of edible product". It should be noted that, since drying involves the loss of water, the nutritional values of 100 grams of fresh food refer to 1000 grams of dried mushrooms.

Properties of mushrooms: they strengthen the immune system and fight cholesterol

The properties of mushrooms can vary considerably depending on the species. However, some of them are common to all mushrooms. Let's see what they are.

"First of all, mushrooms are low in calories, rich in water, and low in fat, which makes them a suitable food for all those who want to lose weight or follow a low-fat diet. Even the fiber content, acting as a satiating factor, is useful in low-calorie diets", suggests the interviewee.

It should be remembered that fiber is very important in regulating intestinal functionality and transit, so the fungus can be of considerable help for those suffering from intestinal dysfunctions.

Another important property of mushrooms is to significantly support the immune system, carrying out important antibacterial properties. For this reason they are recommended during the change of season between summer and autumn, perhaps as part of a detox diet, not surprisngly their typical "flowering" season, precisely to strengthen the immune system and help the body to defend itself better: "Ths action is mainly carried out by the polysaccharides that mushrooms contain, which are able to rebalance the immune system, both when it is hyperstimulated by allergies or inflammation, and when it is in deficient conditions, caused for example by chronic infections". The immunostimulating action is also enhanced by the presence of selenium, capable of stimulating the production of cytokines by leukocytes, specifically responsible for the immune response to infections. The good selenium content is also beneficial for hair, nails and teeth, also having antioxidant properties.

Among the properties of mushrooms, the positive action on the nervous system and on the metabolism of proteins, lipids and carbohydrates should also be mentioned, thanks to the rich content of B vitamins. Useful in preventing and countering anemia and its annoying symptoms such as weakness, headaches and digestive problems, thanks to the good iron content, mushrooms are also able to counteract the accumulation of bad cholesterol in the blood vessels, thus helping to prevent problems related to circulation. The high calcium content also protects the bones, helping to prevent the onset of various diseases affecting the skeletal system, primarily osteoporosis. Thanks to the richness in potassium, "mushrooms have a protective action against the heart and the circulatory system in general, regulating blood pressure, as well as an improvement of memory and cognitive functions". They also contain natural insulin and enzymes that help the body break down the sugars and starch contained in food.

Some constituents of mushrooms support liver and pancreatic function, thus promoting the production of insulin in a natural way: "they can therefore be eaten in case of hyperglycemia and even diabetes, although in the latter case, especially if the patient is treated with an insulin, their intake must be carefully evaluated by a professional. Finally, the presence of antioxidants, useful against cellular aging, should be remembered", concludes the nutritionist Evangelisti about the properties of mushrooms.

MUSHROOMS IN THE KITCHEN: ALL USES

The properties of mushrooms from a health point of view are very interesting, however, the aspect that interests most is their gastronomic value. Certainly, the most popular is the porcini , fleshy and very fragrant, suitable for the preparation of sauces or for frying, which can be harvested between the end of summer and the beginning of autumn, typically near oaks and chestnuts.

The cardoncello, with its large and fleshy hat, is also very appreciated and excellent when roasted on the plate. The champignon is instead a cultivated mushroom, therefore available all year round and suitable for the most varied preparations.

Mushrooms are well suited for the preparation of numerous savory dishes. In addition to being enjoyed as such, for example fried or baked in the oven, mushrooms can also be used in small quantities, as an addition to sauces or to a meat or vegetable broth, making these preparations much tastier and tastier. The famous mushroom risotto is very well known, as well as roasted and grilled mushrooms. More innovative, but equally tasty, is the warm salad of kamut and champignon mushrooms, as well as the bresaola rolls with mushroom carpaccio and the mushroom and potato soup.

HOW TO STORE MUSHROOMS

"Since mushroom picking is limited only to certain periods of the year, which also depend on climatic conditions, the mushroom is a food that can hardly be consumed fresh, which is why, after harvesting, they must be stored correctly" , specifies the interviewee. There are several conservation methods, useful in order to maintain their nutritional properties. The best known, applied very often to porcini mushrooms, is drying, which consists of evaporating the water contained in the mushroom. This process is a good preservation method as the nutrients are preserved; the only trick is to necessarily rehydrate the mushroom before consumption, soaking it in water until the soft consistency returns. Another technique is preservation in oil, which consists in boiling the mushrooms for a few minutes in equal parts of oil and vinegar and placing them in jars completely covered with the cooking liquid.

However, the nutritionist observes that this method, "in addition to causing the loss of part of the nutrients in the cooking liquid, can be dangerous for the possible development of food botulism, so you must be very careful, remembering that the presence of bubbles in the jar 'air is an indication of danger". Finally, another method of conservation is freezing, much safer, to be carried out after a thorough washing to remove the earth. In this case, to avoid possible flaking it is advisable to place the mushrooms in the lower part of the freezer and cook the mushrooms while they are still frozen, in order not to lose the nutrients during defrosting.

CONTRAINDICATIONS: WHEN CAN IT BE DANGEROUS TO CONSUME MUSHROOMS?

The contraindications relating to mushrooms basically refer to any allergies, risk of intoxication and possible consumption of poisonous mushrooms, and excess quantities. In addition to deriving from the ingestion of poisonous mushrooms, mushroom poisoning can also occur following the consumption of toxic mushrooms, but also simply spoiled or infested ones. In fact, fungi are organisms particularly subject to infestations by parasites and bacteria which are then responsible, in this case, for intoxication. So, what to do to consume them safely? "First of all, if we use fresh mushrooms, we must pay attention when buying, carefully evaluating the external appearance. The fungus must be compact and without dents, traces of mold or rotten parts, a sign that the presence of bacteria or parasites is possible. The same criterion of judgment must of course be applied if you go to gather them directly outdoors, in this case also having the attention not to pick poisonous species (some very similar in appearance to edible ones)", highlights the nutritionist.

The signs of intoxication are always well evident, and typically include, in minor cases:

- ✓ nausea
- ✓ retching
- ✓ diarrhea
- ✓ abdominal pain
- ✓ temperature
- ✓ sweating
- ✓ red spots on the skin.

In severe cases, hallucinations, hypertension, headaches, significant liver damage and, in some cases, even death may appear. Many think that milk has detoxifying power, thus acting as an "antidote" in such cases, but the doctor explains that it is a false belief: "'the only thing you have to do when you recognize the symptoms of mushroom poisoning, is to go to the emergency room to receive the most appropriate care ".

Even mushrooms in oil can be dangerous because, in case of bad conservation, Botox can develop; therefore better not to buy them if we are not absolutely sure of the condition of the product, while, if we want to prepare them ourselves, it is a good idea to carefully wash the mushrooms and blanch them with water and vinegar before placing them in the jar which, of course, must be well sterilized.

Another important recommendation is not to exceed the quantities, and this is due to various factors that affect all species of mushrooms, and therefore also edible ones, in fact: "mushrooms are quite difficult to digest, due to the presence, in their cell wall, chitin, a polysaccharide similar to that which makes up the exoskeleton of insects and, therefore, very difficult to metabolize. Moreover, they tend to easily absorb atmospheric pollution, due to their typical spongy fiber". Finally, that Reishi mushrooms are to be avoided in case of taking anticoagulant, immunosuppressive and antiplatelet drugs.

MEDICINAL MUSHROOMS

In the West, since ancient times, mushrooms have been viewed with suspicion due to some varieties being poisonous, in some cases even deadly (for example Amanita phalloides). In the East, on the other hand, the mushroom is considered a precious therapeutic complement to the diet and for centuries medicinal mushrooms have been used by Traditional Chinese Medicine for the treatment of many diseases (mycotherapy)

In fact, fungi, living in a very hostile environment, in order to survive insects, microbes and temperature changes, must produce various substances including antibiotics, vitamins of group D and B and precious trace elements. Although they all have common properties, each mushroom, depending on the family it belongs to, has, in relation to its chemical composition, a different pharmacological activity. All mushrooms are therefore rich in trace elements, vitamins and immunostimulating substances in general, but each of them has its own peculiarities.

The therapeutic properties of mushrooms can be exploited by humans by consuming them as a preventive food, or by taking them in the form of extracts or tablets or capsules, forms more suitable for people suffering from real pathologies.

They are particularly indicated in the treatment of metabolic pathologies such as diabetes and hypercholesterolemia in general, but also in the metabolic syndrome, a very frequent condition today, related to sedentary lifestyle and obesity and the premise of many other pathologies. Medicinal mushrooms are also specifically indicated in more serious degenerative diseases, such as cancer. In these conditions they can play an interesting complementary role and enhancement of official therapies, such as chemotherapy and radiotherapy. Among the more than 400 mushrooms in which medicinal properties have been recognized, in this article we report the 12 most important, whose properties reported here are supported by numerous studies. They are also the easiest to find on the market and at a reasonable price.

THE 12 MEDICINAL MUSHROOMS:

- ✓ Agaricus blazei murrill
- ✓ Auricularia auricula-judae
- ✓ Coprinus comatus
- ✓ Cordyceps sinensis
- ✓ Coriolus versicolor
- ✓ Ganoderma lucidum (Reishi)
- ✓ Hericium erinaceus
- ✓ Maitake (Grifola frondosa)
- ✓ Shiitake (Lentinus edodes)
- ✓ Pleurotus ostreatus
- ✓ Polyporus umbrellatus
- ✓ Poria cocos

AGARICUS BLAZEI MURRILL (ABM)

Agaricus Blazei Murrill Mushroom Also known by the Japanese name of Himematsutake, Agaricus Blazei Murrill (ABM) is a mushroom originating from the mountainous regions of

Piedade, Brazil. 30 years ago, in the 90s, some epidemiologists, studying the native population of the Piedade near San Paolo, noticed that the rate of diseases in this region was extremely low and correlated it to the regular consumption of this mushroom in the diet.

Subsequent experiments conducted in Japan on mice found that this fungus resulted in a significant activation of the immune system in excess of that attributed to shiitake, maitake, reishi and other "medicinal" mushrooms. This fungus has been attributed to the prevention of neoplastic diseases, diabetes, hyperlipidemia, atherosclerosis and chronic hepatitis.

AURICULARIA AURICULA-JUDAE

Auricularia auricula-judae mushroom is an edible sessile mushroom, commonly ear-shaped, brownish red, gelatinous, elastic, with a sweet taste and imperceptible odor. It grows on dead trees or parts of trees and can reach a size of 3 to 10 cm.

This fungus has an immunostabilising effect, determines an increase in the number of white blood cells. Rich in adenosine, it promotes blood circulation without inducing hemorrhages, but hinders platelet aggregation, reduces hyperlipidemia and therefore prevents thrombotic phenomena, atherosclerosis, and obstruction of blood vessels without attacking collagen and thus preserving its integrity. The inclusion of Auricularia in the diet favors a decrease in bad cholesterol (LDL), without altering the values of good cholesterol (HDL).

It is able to dissolve already existing atheromatous plaques. It is a useful mushroom for the prevention of cardiovascular diseases, resolving circulatory alterations, especially in the legs, in peripheral venous insufficiency (PVD peripherical vascular disease). It increases the activity of SOD, stimulating the antioxidant and anti-inflammatory activity. Activates the metabolism of lactic acid after physical effort. It strengthens all the mucous membranes and has, in general, a humectant effect on them, therefore it is useful in dry cough, pharyngitis, sinusitis, but also in chronic colitis with constipation. It has antidiabetic properties attributable to the creation of a viscous mass induced by the hydration of its fibers which slows down intestinal transit and therefore also the absorption of sugars.

COPRINUS COMATUS

Coprinus comatus mushroom is an edible mushroom common all over the world which, with aging, takes on a bluish color and is therefore called the "ink fungus". There are more than 100 ink mushrooms and they are found on rich, non-fertilized soils, on meadows, fields and gardens and are very common in our latitudes. It has a 3-6 cm cap, oval to bell-shaped at the top, a thin and elongated stem that can reach up to 20 cm. It is mostly white and covered with dense scales. with age the cap opens and takes on a blackish color and withers.

Coprinus contains many minerals, the main ones being potassium and vanadium, but also calcium, iron, copper and zinc. It is rich in amino acids including 8 essential and from 20 to 40% proteins, vitamins C, D, E and group B (especially Niacir). Thanks to the vanadium content, Coprinus comatus is a fungus that targets the endocrine pancreas and its diseases: type I and II diabetes. Vanadium, in this peculiar phytocomplex, is responsible for the antidiabetic effect that manifests itself, at the peripheral level, through the sensitization of cellular receptors for insulin, and at central level with the revitalization with regenerative capacity of the islets of Langerahans (pancreatic beta cells) residual and, to date, no side effects have been reported, unlike what has been reported with the use of the single mineral vanadium.

Studies on the use of this mushroom have shown a fast (90') and persistent reduction in blood sugar (6 hours) characterizing it as a real oral hypoglycemic agent without however the side effects of hypoglycemic drugs. It helps digestion and assists weight reduction with the same caloric-energy intake. It also improves blood circulation and prevents atherosclerosis by helping to dissolve atheromatous plaques and make arterial walls more elastic. An antitumor action has been noted for this fungus especially at the level of connective and supporting tissues.

CORDYCEPS SINENSIS

Cordyceps sinensis fungus, also known as Dong Chong Xia Cao, or Tochukaso, is a parasitic fungus of a moth of the Hepialidae family, of which it progressively invades the larva sunk in the ground. It originates from the Tibetan plateau (Qinghai region) between 3,000 and 5,000 meters above sea level. In Traditional Chinese Medicine (TCM) it is considered the mushroom of potency, as it confers vigor, endurance and willpower.

According to TCM it supports the kidneys which store vital energy. Cordyceps helps to regenerate the body after diseases by providing energy to the body and mind. It stimulates the immune system through the stimulation of Peyer's plaques and the activation of macrophages and NKs. Contains cordycepin which has an effect similar to antibiotics, limits the growth of Clostridium perfringens and Clostridium paraputricum (anaerobic and acidifying pathogenic bacteria that favor the onset of degenerative pathologies), but does not destroy good microorganisms, such as bifidobacterium and lactobacilli, preserving intestinal flora.

It has a stimulating function on the sexual apparatus, on the production of sex hormones and on the neurological system involved in reproduction and sexual performance. It has the same effect as an aphrodisiac. It can be helpful in depression when accompanied by a lack of motivation and willpower, fear, anxiety and a feeling of emptiness. Some authors argue that its stimulating effect on hormonal release from the adrenal glands works in managing symptoms of stress.

Using Cordyceps reduces LDL and VLDL cholesterol and increases HDL good cholesterol. Increase your corticosteroid level 1 hour after taking. At the renal level it protects the glomeruli: it hinders the formation of glomerulosclerosis (cell proliferation of the mesangium) linked to an increase in LDL. It is a mushroom with an excellent tropism for the liver: after 25 days of taking the extract in mice it was possible to notice a 36% increase in Kupfer cells compared to controls (dose dependent mode). From this point of view it can be very useful in the treatment of hepatic fibrosis and forms of viral hepatitis B and C. It is a widely used mushroom for athletes for its ability to restore muscle and improve cardio-circulatory function.

CORIOLUS VERSICOLOR

Coriolus versicolor medicinal mushroom is a mushroom of varying color considered inedible due to its woody texture and bitter taste, which grows all over the world on live or dead trunks and stumps. For centuries this mushroom has been used in Traditional Chinese Medicine as an anticancer drug and in the 1980s the Japanese government approved the use of its extracts which are currently among the best-selling cancer drugs in this country.

In the "Compendium of Chinese Materia Medica" more than 120 strains of Coriolus versicolor are recorded; its use is indicated to detoxify, strengthen the body, increase energy and stimulate immune functions. Also, in TCM it is clinically indicated for various cancers, for chronic hepatitis and for infections of the upper respiratory, urinary and digestive tract.

In the last 30 years it has also been deeply studied in the West both in vivo and in vitro and in animal models. In vitro, its extracts have been found to be effective in activating T and B lymphocytes and monocytes / macrophages, bone marrow cells, Natural Killer and activated Killer lymphocytes and in increasing the expression of particular cytokines, Tumor Necrosis Factor and interference. In vivo studies revealed that the aqueous extracts of Coriolus do not exert visible effects on normal people, while they are able to restore an immunological response in immunosuppressed patients, with stimulation of complement and specific cytokines and interferons, increasing the patient's resistance. to bacterial or fungal infections when administered intraperitoneally.

Im Oriente, numerous clinical trials have been carried out on the activity of this medicinal mushroom, in most of which the oral administration of Coriolus versicolor whole mushroom or biomass (mycelium) has resulted in a significant increase in the patient's response and quality of life. oncological. The advantage of this supportive therapy is the efficacy of oral administration and the possibility of long-term therapy as it is very well tolerated. The effect of this fungus in inhibiting telomerase activity and consequent promotion of tumor regression is very important.

GANODERMA LUCIDUM

Ganoderma lucidum reishi mushroom, also known as Reishi and Ling Zhi, is an inedible mushroom with a woody consistency and a characteristic glossy appearance, hence its name. In the East it is known as the "mushroom of immortality" or "mushroom of 10,000 years" or even "herb of spiritual power" and there are documented reports of its use in China several centuries before the birth of Christ. It is an adaptogenic fungus able to exert a general stimulus of the organism and an anti-aging support. It is counted among the 10 most effective natural therapeutic substances, as it is very rich in bioactive molecules: polysaccharides, triterpenes, mineral salts (iron, zinc, manganese, magnesium, potassium, germanium and calcium), B vitamins, 17 amino acids including all the essentials, sterols and cortisone-like substances, adenosine and guanosine with anti-platelet effect, muscle relaxant (skeletal muscle) and sedative of the CNS.

Triterpenes are mainly responsible for the adaptogenic properties of the fungus, while germanium exerts an oxygenating action, analgesic effects and stimulates the production of interferon. The spores of the mushroom are particularly rich in triterpenes, while the mycelium (biomass) of enzymes and the whole mushroom of beta-glucans. Depending on the action sought, the part of the mushroom (however in its entirety) that most satisfies it must be chosen. The spores will therefore be used for a greater anti-allergic, antihistamine and anti-inflammatory action, the whole mushroom for the immunomodulating action and the mycelium or spores for the anti-inflammatory and anti-aging action.

Given its sedation of the CNS, Reishi will be the mushroom of choice even in cases of anxiety and insomnia. Ganoderma Lucidum exerts a toning action on the heart and cardiovascular system both directly, as a rhythm for the heart and as an ACE-inhibitor effect on hypertension, and indirectly acting as an anti-platelet and cholesterol-lowering agent.

This mushroom also has strong anti-allergic and anti-inflammatory properties, thanks to the modulation of the immune system and the presence of substances with cortisone and antihistamine action. The intake of Reishi determines a net increase in the immune response in immunosuppressed and neoplastic patients and a better management of the side effects of chemo and radiotherapy. It works very well in prevention, in particular for viral infections and exerts a strong antioxidant action, protecting cell structures from oxidative damage. It is also helpful in the case of diabetes, since the presence of fibers reduces the enteric absorption of glucose and the ganoderic acids A, B and C determine a better peripheral utilization of glucose and a stimulation of hepatic glucose metabolism. Finally, Ganoderma Lucidum possesses hepatoprotective properties in particular in inflammatory hepatopathies and in hepatotoxicity due to myotherapy, where it stimulates detoxification and restores liver function.

HERICIUM HERINACEUS

Hericium herinaceus mushroom is a very rare mushroom, considered a delicacy even if a bit tough. It develops preferably on live oak trees, or on beech, walnut, plane trees and other broad-leaved trees. It grows on the trunk to a height of about 3-4 meters. The fruiting body resembles the head of a monkey so in Asia it is called "monkey head".

Hericium contains numerous minerals (potass um, zinc, iron, germanium, selenium and phosphorus), all essential amino acids, immunomodulating polysaccharides (beta glucans) and antitumor effect (FII 1- FIII2b), ericenones, erinacins and a factor similar to Nerve Growth Factor (NGF). It is a fungus that works mainly on ectodermal tissues (mucous membranes and nervous system).

Its therapeutic effects are expressed at the level of the gastric and intestinal mucosa, as it has a regenerating action of the mucous membranes, and can be very useful in the treatment of heartburn, gastritis, gastric and duodenal ulcers, chronic inflammation of the gastric mucosa also consequent to chemo and radiotherapy, ulcerative colitis and Crohn's disease.

The presence of a substance similar to NGF stimulates the synthesis of myelin and the reconstruction of nerve fibers. Its effects on the nervous system are multiple and articulated; its use is useful in the treatment of anxiety, stress, mnemonic deficits and insomnia. Clinical studies have found encouraging results in the treatment of multiple sclerosis and Alzheimer's disease. The presence of immunomodulating polysaccharides and its tropism for the epithelia and the nervous system makes it useful in the treatment of dermatological problems of psychosomatic, allergic or food intolerance (dermatitis and neurodermatitis) derivation. The ability of this fungus to regenerate the intestinal mucosa and restore a correct intestinal flora make it useful in the treatment of dysbiosis with consequent high inflammatory rations of the mucosa (Leaky Gut Syndrome).

MAITAKE

Maitake (scientific name: Grifola frondosa) is a Japanese mushroom that grows mainly in autumn, near oaks, horse chestnuts and beech trees and develops with a porous and branched structure with brown-gray caps. It is a very rare, very good and very precious mushroom, which was once exchanged for equal weight in silver (1kg of maitake for 1kg of silver).

Contains mineral salts, amino acids, B vitamins, precursors of vitamin D2 (ergosterol), polysaccharides (fraction D) and antioxidant enzymes. The administration of the mushroom powder has shown hypoglycemic effects, corrective of hypertension and hypertriglyceridemia. It is therefore very useful in the treatment of the metabolic syndrome.

Promotes the elimination of bile acids and triglycerides through the faeces. It acts as a natural regulator of lipid metabolism avoiding the accumulation of fat in the liver. It is very useful in the treatment of liver statosis. It reduces hypercholesterolemia by keeping the HDL good cholesterol values constant.

It counteracts increases in body weight and has a marked antidiabetic action (non-insulin-dependent diabetes II) which is expressed through an increase in the sensitivity of insulin cell receptors; it also promotes an increase in the number of insulin receptors by increasing the body's ability to recognize and metabolise glucose.

Known for its immunostimulation effects attributed to the D-polysaccharide fraction, when administered orally it increases the macrophage activity, number and efficacy of Natural Killer cells and cytotoxic T lymphocytes. In Japan it is used, in dosages from 3 to 7 g per day, for the prevention of neoplastic disease, as an immunostimulant in cancer patients and as a support to chemo and radiotherapy.

SHIITAKE

Shiitake (scientific name: Lentinus edodes) is a mushroom that comes from the East, widespread in ancient China even before rice cultivation and for about hundreds of years it is an integral part of the Japanese diet. Its name derives from "Shii" (oak) and "Take" (mushroom) because it grows spontaneously in the trunks of these trees.

In mycotherapy Shiitake is mainly used in the treatment of blood pressure changes and as an immunoregulator. Useful in cases of migraine and tinnitus, related to circulatory alterations. It obtains   excellent   results   in   the   treatment   of hypercholesterolemia, reducing total cholesterol and raising the values of good HDL cholesterol, thanks to the presence of choline and erythroadenin which regulates the level of fat in the blood through an improvement in blood circulation (increases the peripheral resistance, regulates heart rate and power).

It acts in the prevention and treatment of atherosclerosis, helping to clean the vessel walls of sediments, which is the cause of the formation of atherosclerosis plaques. The vitamin D contained in it promotes the metabolism of calcium and contributes to the removal of any calcium deposits in the arterial walls.

It has an alkalizing effect and is effective in the treatment of hyperuricemia and gout. Lentinan, a high molecular weight polysaccharide, contained both in the fungus and in the mycelium, is used in Japan intratumorally in the treatment of stomach tumors. It is an immunomodulating agent and is used a lot in children and young people in case of weakening of the immune system due to viral diseases, allergies, infections and bronchial and joint inflammation. The mycelium contains another glycoprotein (LEM) with antitumor activity such as Lentinan.

PLEUROTUS OSTREATUS

Pleurotus ostreatus also called oyster, is the most common among the pleural mushrooms, it is found in autumn and winter in the northern temperate zones. It grows on dead deciduous wood (poplar, willow, mulberry, etc.). It can be found isolated or, more frequently, in groups, even bushy, forming the typical cascade with the caps positioned on a shelf. It is an excellent edible mushroom after prolonged cooking to soften the firm and tenacious structure of the meat.

This fungus has important actions in the body, especially on the digestive system and as a regulator of blood cholesterol levels. Pleurotus ostreatus contains: a high percentage of proteins, of which 8 essential amino acids (all except tryptophan), B vitamins (B1, B2, B3, B5, B7), vitamin C and PP and mineral salts (calcium, magnesium, iron, copper, manganese, phosphorus, potassium, selenium, sodium and zinc). In addition, Pleurotus contains several bioactive compounds that are responsible for the immunomodulating effects, the antibacterial, antiviral, anti-inflammatory, antitumor action that numerous studies have attributed to it: beta-glucans and glycoproteins, lovastatin, ostreolysin, laccase, D-glucose oxidase, ribonuclease, dimeric lectins, 9 kD peptide with ribonuclease activity, palmitic and linoleic acid.

The main bioactive substances, attributable to the beneficial effect of this fungus on the body, are dietary fibers, B vitamins, numerous antioxidants and lovastatin. Dietary fibers make Pleurotus ostreatus an excellent prebiotic; these substances are not absorbed by the body but are used by the intestinal flora. They also have interesting nutritional properties in subjects with diabetes, metabolic syndrome, systemic acidosis, obesity and allergy.

Containing a natural statin (Lovastatin) it has a strong anti-cholesterol action. Pleorotus can be used, not only as a food and drug, but also industrially to absorb and digest oil slick, possibly dispersed in water; it can also digest plastic containers.

Some studies attribute Pleorotus, taken in high doses, to the ability to increase testosterone and estrogen levels, thus protecting bone, brain and cardiovascular structures, as well as reducing bothersome symptoms of menopause.

POLYPORUS UMBRELLATUS

Polyporus umbellatus is an edible mushroom that grows in Europe and Asia in "clumps" of considerable size and weight, and is characterized by a sweet, slightly fresh taste and a neutral smell. According to Traditional Chinese Medicine, this fungus has an effect on the spleen, kidneys and bladder. In TCM it is used to move the stagnation of liquids, therefore for edema and as a diuretic, even in case of painful urination and in general in all bladder dysfunctions, from infections to cancer and kidney (nephritis).

In infections it acts as an antibiotic, while the anticancer effect is linked to the inhibition of DNA replication in cancer cells. Contains polysaccharides, polypeptides, minerals (calcium, potassium, iron, manganese, copper and zinc) B vitamins (especially Biotin), and secondary metabolites (including ergosterine and alpha hydroxy tetracosanoic acid).

The intake of Polyporus increases diuresis with the elimination of sodium, but not potassium, so that the neuro-muscular function is protected. Has anti-hypertensive effect; promotes the reabsorption of edema; improves the epidermal structure with a positive effect on skin diseases especially if linked to an overload of the lymphatic system; relaxes muscle tissue; strengthens the respiratory system; strengthens the lymphatic system by hindering the accumulation of liquids and therefore stagnation; strengthens the heart, promotes blood circulation by helping to clean the blood vessels; by cleaning the lymphatic system, it exerts an anti-tumor prevention effect, but also detoxifies after chemotherapy; in the treatment of bladder cancer showed a reduction in relapses of 50%. Clinical studies have highlighted the usefulness of this mushroom in the combined treatment of lung cancer and leukemia.

PORIA COCOS

Poria cocos is a distinctive underground potato-like fungus that grows underground as a root parasite of pine and other conifers. It is widespread in wooded areas and near conifers in northern China.

Traditionally it is harvested from the ground in late summer, then dried for a long time until the surface appears rough; the consistency is soft and has a sweet or neutral flavor.

It is believed to be able to purify the body, improve the function of the spleen and consequently, according to Traditional Chinese Medicine, to calm the mind. It is included in numerous traditional tonic compositions useful in case of lack of appetite, diarrheal stools, nervousness and insomnia.

Cases of schizophrenia have been reported treated with high doses of the fungus. Some scholars have compared its antidepressant effect to that of Prozac. If taken as a supplement it could prove useful to calm anxiety, to facilitate sleep but also to reduce the incessant whirlwind of thoughts. Poria cocos also has a sedative effect on the cardiovascular level and is indicated in case of tachycardia, palpitations and insomnia of cardiac origin. Promotes diuresis and the removal of toxins that stagnate with the accumulation of fluids in the body.

Poria Cocos is also a valid ally for the immune system, as it stimulates the immune defences and is suitable for those who are in a state of physical debilitation.

DEADLY POISONOUS MUSHROOMS

THE GREAT MURDERERS

mushrooms can kill

In a mushroom it is essential to carefully observe the stem, the cap and the hymenium. The stem supports the cap.

The cap is covered on the top by a skin called the cuticle (more or less separable). The hymenium is the underside of the cap and contains the spores. It is the fertile part of the fungus and in the vast majority of cases it consists of gills (fungus on the left) or a "sponge" (tubes and pores), as in the fungus on the right.

Each fungal family is divided into groups. Each group into genera. Each genus into species. The species indicates the single mushroom, it is its first name. Its surname is not like that of the family for people, but that of the genus. In mycological dictionaries, mushrooms (remember? Actually, we should say carpophores) are listed in alphabetical order by surname and name (genus and species. In the meantime, many years have passed and the classifications have greatly differentiated and expanded. Virtually every mycological school adopts its own classification. However, the fundamentals do not change.

Amanite are medium and large sized mushrooms, with a slender and elegant, typical habit, and a very varied color. From pure white (Virosa, Verna, Solitaria) to dirty-olive white (Phalloide) to deep orange (Caesarea) to bright red (Muscaria) to brown (Panterina). They all have three elements that identify them with certainty as amanite: the volva, the ring and the white lamellae.

If you find a mushroom that doesn't seem to have a volva, don't trust it yet: see if it has the ring and especially the color of the lamellae. If the ring has it and at the same time the blades are white IT'S AN AMANITA: LEAVE IT THERE!

Cortinari are not good mushrooms (with one exception), almost always bitter, ugly to look at. They include several toxic species. Orellanus is the most devious and dangerous of the deadly poisonous mushrooms. Therefore:

RECOGNIZE IT NOW AND LEAVE IT THERE!

HOW TO RECOGNIZE THEM

We just picked up a mushroom. How to exclude with absolute certainty that it is an amanita or a cortinari?

First, let's flip the mushroom and look at its hymenium. All four deadly poisonous mushrooms belong to the Agaricaceae family and feature a reed hymenium. So if this is not lamellar, the mushroom is not part of the quartet. We are not yet safe from even serious poisoning if we eat it, but at least we will not die from it. Here, then, that with a simple gesture we are able to exclude that the mushroom we have caught is one of the four killers. However, there is a big drawback: the vast majority of edible mushrooms belong to the Agaricaceae family, giving up which practically renounces to collect mushrooms. It is therefore necessary to isolate the infamous quartet in a more restricted grouping than the whole family and that is their genus (that of the amanite and that of the cortinari). The keys to do this are indicated in the central body of the article.

There is no lover of nature who has not come across mushrooms, discreet and somewhat mysterious inhabitants of these places during his strolls along woods, clearings and pastures. They seem to appear almost out of nowhere: yesterday they weren't there and today the forest is full of them. They look like plants, but they are not, as they lack the chlorophyll function. They feed on organic substances as occurs in the animal world, without however belonging to it. We stop here because this is a chat between friends which, if read carefully, is equivalent to a life insurance, and not a mycological essay. A minimum of terminology, to understand each other, however, it will be necessary to introduce it. We will do it in small doses, in the right column. However, it should be noted that what we commonly call a mushroom is actually a carpophore, the gigantic "fruit" of that tiny "plant" which is the mycelium. To be picky, by mushroom we should mean the plant plus the fruit, that is, mycelium and carpophore together. Of course, we will not do it here: mushroom we commonly say and mushroom we will write.

THE DEADLY POISONOUS MUSHROOMS

Every year someone dies because they ate poisonous mushrooms they didn't recognize. Generally, it is not about being inexperienced, at their first outings, but being ignorant. The inexperienced are careful not to consume mushrooms they do not know. At risk, however, are those who have been looking for mushrooms for some time and eat them quietly, based on often mistaken beliefs. Hence their ignorance. One of these beliefs, very dangerous, is that the mushrooms of a certain area are all good because you have never heard of a poisoning in those parts. They are unaware that at any moment the wind can carry Amanita Verna spores near a field mushroom farm. An example? My friend Onofrio. Behind his little house in Bugnara he gathers at the foot of old olive trees abundant piopparelli and any other fungus that takes root, convinced that a poisonous mushroom cannot grow on an olive tree. I tried in vain to make him change his mind, even showing him a book on mycology, but I could not shake his conviction gained over years and years of gathering and eating. I really hope for him that the poisonous clitocybe olearia never takes root at the foot of those plants.

An amanita cannot take root on a mushroom farm, but can be nearby. And if the harvest is not a refreshing walk, but a frenetic race made at dawn or even in the dark to arrive before the others and perhaps hearing the noise of another hunter behind him, here is all this is collected, that it is white and round. Quickly and almost without looking, while on the contrary one should observe very carefully. So in the plastic bag (a collector of this type will not use a basket) together with the champignons there ends up some Amanita Verna or Phalloides, two of the four great killers.

THE FOUR GREAT MURDERERS

A minimum of prudence and common sense, observing the simple indications of this chat, is equivalent to a life insurance for those who go for mushrooms because there are only four BIG ASSASSINS. Here they are:

Amanita Phalloides

Slender mushroom generally olive colo~ed but which can vary towards white. Sagging ring. Wide volva

Amanita Verna

Fungus very similar to the phalloid, except for the white color. It is a spring species. They can also be found in autumn, but more than late Verna, they are probably white Phalloides. They are the cause of deadly poisonings in those who believe they have collected field mushrooms.

Amanita Virosa

White mushroom like Verna. The cap, however, contrary to this and the phalloid does not become flattened as an adult, but remains campanulate. It has a floppy ring and a fluffy stem.

Cortinarius Orellanus

He is the only one of the four great killers who is not of the Amanita genus. No volva, no ring, no white gills: they are rusty red like the cap. The stem, initially yellow, soon takes on the typical rust color due to the color of the spores. Contrary to the elegant Amanitas, it is in short, an ugly mushroom.

We have given the name of great killers to these four mushrooms because those who eat them are very likely to die from them. First of all, because the poison of a single specimen is sufficient to kill. Secondly, because the symptoms of poisoning are late (no earlier than seven to eight hours for amanite and even two weeks for Cortinarius Orellanus) and make the first, simpler and, if timely, effective remedy against poisonings useless: gastric lavage. Finally, because the malaise is not due to the body's reaction to toxic substances, but to the malfunctioning of organs that are already severely damaged. Paradoxically, the mushrooms which in addition to amanitins and orellanin also contain other toxic substances are less dangerous because the latter will produce immediate symptoms that will allow prompt medical intervention. The poison of the four deadly fungi penetrates into the liver (mainly the amanitins) and kidney (mainly the orellanins) cells and destroy them with a very rapid chain process.

THE AMANITES

Three of these "great killers" are part of the Amanita genus and one of them the Cortinarius genus. Both genera have absolutely clear identification keys. The purpose of this article is to provide a certain criterion for identifying these two genera in order to exclude all species from our table as a whole. It is true that by doing so, one renounces a priori the excellent Amanita Caesarea and the excellent Cortinarius Praestans, which are easily recognizable, but it is equally true that those who want to learn to recognize mushrooms need time to observe, compare and reflect. Recognizing an Amanita Caesarea or a Cortinarius Praestans is very easy, but there will be time and way for them, while learning to recognize an Amanita and a cortinario as such is so much more important and fundamental that, frankly, in a chat like this, we do not feel like giving the slightest exception to the rule:

RECOGNIZE AN AMANITA AND A CORTINARY IMMEDIATELY AND LEAVE THEM THERE.

AMANITA CAESAREA

When you come across a developed specimen with a very evident typical color like that of Archenzo's photo, the exception could be made, but this is not always the case. The immature specimen that can be glimpsed between the leaves, for example, due to the still intact veil is completely white.

There are three elements that identify the Amanitas:

the volva, the ring and the white blades

THE VOLVA

The volva is a residue of the general veil, that is, of the thin membrane that envelops the fungus in the initial stage, making it similar to an egg. The volva looks like a hood with the opening upwards from which the stem of the mushroom emerges.

CAUTION

In two cases we may not notice the volva:

1) If we cut the stem instead of plucking the whole mushroom (the volva remains in the ground)

2) If the volva is inconspicuous and appears not as a hood but as a simple enlargement of the stem.

Amanites, apart from the rare and small volvaria, are the only mushrooms to have a volva, therefore: if a mushroom has a volva it is an Amanita: leave it there.

If it seems to you that a mushroom does not have a volva, do not trust it yet: see if it has a ring.

THE RING

The ring is a residue of the secondary veil that is initially found under the cap, to protect the hymenium, the fertile part of the fungus. As the spores reach maturity, the veil exhausts its function and therefore falls. In most cases it disappears completely, without leaving a trace, but in some species, as in all amanitas, it detaches from the lower edge of the cap but not from the stem, thus forming the ring. A showy ring is typical of the Amanita genus, but the genera Lepiota, Psalliota, Armillaria and Pholiota are also provided with it, therefore it represents an alarm bell, not an identifier of amanite, as is the case for the volva.

THE WHITE REEDS

The white lamellae are a very important identification element. ATTENTION: not off-white, cream or havana: WHITE!

Amanites, even in mature specimens, always have white gills. If this were taken into account, many poisonings would be avoided. The amanitas, in fact, are often taken for champignons. If during the harvest the stem is cut, instead of plucking the whole mushroom, the volva remains in the ground. The ring does not make you suspicious, because even the field mushrooms have it and so the last chance to avoid making a fatal mistake is to observe the color of the lamellae. Only in the Amanita the gills remain white even in the adult mushroom. In champignons they quickly become dirty white, then hazel, havana and dark brown.

CAUTION

VOLVA = AMANITA (or volvaria)

RING + WHITE REEDS = AMANITA

THE CORTINARIES

Cortinari are not good mushrooms (with one exception, Praestans), almost always bitter, ugly to look at. They include several toxic species. The Orellanus is the most devious and dangerous of them and by far the worst of the big four killers. We have always wondered how it can be that someone thinks to eat a mushroom of this aspect and moreover of bad taste! The cortinari have neither volva nor ring. When young, the cap and hymenium are wrapped in a single veil, called curtain (hence the name) which then disappears, without forming a ring.

The color of the stem is not reddish, as it might seem, but yellowish. To be sure, just cut the stem lengthwise. The rust color is given by the spores of the fungus that stain it. Look at them well, those rusty red mushrooms and store them in your memory and .... stay away! Do not collect anything that even vaguely resembles it. And if by doing so you neglect some Inocybe and some Hebeloma, better this way because they are not tasty mushrooms and many of them are toxic. Therefore:

IF A MUSHROOM HAS A CURTAIN; IT IS A
CORTINARY: LEAVE IT THERE.

The Praestans represents, for the cortinari, what the Caesarea represents for the amanite: the excellent exception. Cortinarius Praestans is also easily recognizable by its robust size which differentiates it from the others. It is the only one with a full, pot-bellied stem.

BEWARE: of Cortinarius Praestans and Amanita Caesarea we have only spoken for completeness of information, but:

NO CORTINARY AND NO ANAMITA MUST BE CONSUMED WITHOUT THE PREVENTIVE OPINION OF A CERTIFIED EXPERT! (Unless you have already gained an excellent theoretical-practical preparation, but in this case this article will not even be read).

THE POISONOUS MUSHROOMS WITH FAST TOXIC ACTION

Mushrooms contain a mix of toxic substances combined with each other. They are divided into a fast-acting and a slow-acting group, much more dangerous than the first, as we have seen. In fact, when intestinal pains, nausea, vomiting, copious sweating, state of agitation, fainting, violent reaction to alcohol arise immediately, it is possible to intervene promptly by eliminating the fungus with vomiting, purges and, in the most serious cases, with gastric lavage, as well as with appropriate hepatoprotective therapy.

POISONOUS MUSHROOMS

non-fatal (if you rush to the hospital)

Amanita Muscaria POISONOUS MUSHROOM

Amanita Aureola POISONOUS MUSHROOM

Amanita Panterina POISONOUS MUSHROOM

For this reason, paradoxically, between two mushrooms that contain the first amanitine (in the plural, because there are at least five) plus muscarine or mycoatropin, substances that already after an hour, cause symptoms of gastrointestinal poisoning and nervous disorders, and according to that it contains the same quantity of amanitins and only those (in one amanita Phalloides there are enough to kill a person weighing 60 kilos) the most dangerous is the latter. After having said about the four most dangerous mushrooms, those to which I have given the nickname of great killers because they attack the liver and kidneys in silence and the first symptoms of poisoning occur after a long time, when these organs are already gone, let's talk about poisonous mushrooms with fast toxic action. There are so many. The most dangerous are Amanita Muscaria, Amanita Aureola and Amanita Panterina.

Amanita Muscaria

The classic red mushroom with white dots. In reality these are not pigments, but warts. It causes neurotropic poisoning.

Amanita Aureola

The most dangerous of the three. Not because it is more toxic than the others, but because it can be confused with Amanita Caesarea, an excellent and sought-after mushroom. The warts can disappear, leaving the color of the cap very similar to that of the Caesarea.

Amanita Panterina

The hazelnut brown color of the cap is characteristic. These mushrooms are also considered to be all three variants of Amanita Muscaria. They are less dangerous than the "big four killers" for three reasons:

1) A single mushroom is not enough to kill. 2) They cause immediate neurotropic poisoning which allows for prompt medical treatment. 3) They are immediately recognizable (almost always) by the warts on the cap.

HALLUCINOGENIC MUSHROOMS - PSILOCYBIN, MAGIC MUSHROOMS

The substance

Hallucinogenic mushrooms grow almost everywhere and are considered the oldest drug known to mankind.

Traditionally, hallucinogenic mushrooms are used for medical and ritual purposes in various places around the world (Southeast Asia, Central America and Latin America). Magic mushrooms contain the psychoactive combinations psilocybin and psilocin. The best known are the psylos, Mexicans and Hawaiians. Hallucinogenic mushrooms can be eaten fresh or dried, but they can also be synthesized into a white powder.

The maximum effect of the mushrooms takes place no earlier than two hours after taking and decreases after 4 - 5 hours.

A particular risk in taking this type of drug is represented by the possible confusion with poisonous mushrooms: for this reason, it is advisable to always keep a specimen of the mushrooms consumed in order to allow their determination.

Warning: ordinary mushrooms sprinkled with LSD are sold on the market and then passed off as hallucinogenic mushrooms!

Freshly harvested mushrooms remain undried for up to a day, after which consumption of spoiled fungal proteins can cause nausea and vomiting.

The effects

Hallucinogenic mushrooms are part of the psychedelic substances and their effects are similar to those of LSD although much less intense. The term derives from the Greek "psyche", soul, and "delos" (clear, evident). In legal texts, police reports and the mass media, "psychedelic" substances are generally defined as hallucinogenic drugs.

In small quantities (between 0.3 and 0.8 g) the mushrooms are stimulating and invigorating, in heavier doses (between 1 and 5 g) the mushrooms are hallucinogenic and produce intense psychedelic effects. Like LSD, mushrooms cause profound changes in consciousness, ego sensation and perception of the surrounding world. Unlike LSD, travel time with mushrooms is generally shorter and easier to manage than LSD. At a high dosage of magic mushrooms or after consuming a mix of mushrooms and alcohol, the danger of a "horror trip" can be higher than with LSD. Psilocybin usually generates a steadily positive mood, and mood swings are less frequent than traveling with LSD. Additionally, psilocybin causes less anxiety in the event that apparently repressed personal conflicts resurface.

The dispersal of the effect and the regeneration after consumption of the mushrooms are considered less traumatic by experienced consumers.

Through the effect of these substances, the brain artificially enters a sort of trance state that normally occurs only in dreams and, despite this, you find yourself in a state of hypervigilance for many hours. Mushrooms intensify and alter your sensory perception and experience intense visual hallucinations. The reality perceived by your eyes is reinterpreted by your brain in different shapes, colors and images. Sounds take on color, objects begin to show their energy. The faster the ideas flow, the harder it becomes to express them orally. The notion of time is lost and it becomes impossible to realize what time it is. Auditory, olfactory, gustatory and tactile sensations are also more intense and in part deeply distorted. Your mood and feelings can change suddenly. A sense of bliss and cheerfulness can suddenly turn into an attack of panic and terror and vice versa.

The experience with these substances is very strong and leaves a lasting impression. The effects of mushrooms are however very related to the dosage ("drug"), the "set" and the "setting".

Risks and secondary effects

Under the influence of fungi, the pupils dilate, the pulse and blood pressure change, the body temperature rises and it is more difficult to breathe. In some cases, you may feel a sense of nausea and vomiting. There may also be disturbances in balance, distortions in the perception of time and space, anxiety and panic.

Sexual desire is often heightened during a psychedelic trip. Erotic games and orgasm are experienced in a new dimension. Increased availability for risky sexual practices (in relation to the transmission of AIDS and hepatitis). It is therefore absolutely necessary that any sexual intercourse under the influence of these drugs be decided first, experimenting with the relative practices in a normal state, taking the necessary precautions to reduce the risk and always with a condom.

If you collect mushrooms in the woods yourself, you risk confusing them with some deadly species.

Magic mushrooms do not cause harm to the body, but in the initial phase of the psychedelic journey, slight disturbances in breathing, heartbeat, changes in blood pressure and sweating following hyperthermia can still occur.

The risks of using magic mushrooms are decidedly on the psychic level and depend on the personality structure of those who use them: thus, while people without serious psychic problems report positive experiences and amazing insights, for people who ponder unsolved problems, for those who have a weak ego or for people who tend to be psychotic, a single trip gone wrong ("horror trip") is enough to have to resort to psychiatric treatment. An excessive frequency of consumption or a too strong dose can also cause these consequences.

If a friend is having a bad trip, try to stay calm and do what you can to calm them down. Take him to a quiet and well-ventilated place, talk to him and reassure him reminding him that the effects of the substance will disappear. However, if those who are high cannot get rid of their delirium, do not hesitate to turn to help. A doctor can administer remedies that will allow for a rapid descent from the effects

THE LIFE CYCLE OF MUSHROOMS

Aculeate: externally equipped with quills, conical or pyramidal asperities similar aspine.

Spore (of spore or of the hymenial apparatus): asperity similar to a sting or a thorn, conical or pyramidal

Adnata: (referring to a lamella) inserted into the stem for most of its height

Alveolus: small cavity, sort of cell for mostly closed.

Alutaceous: pale yellow color tending to incarnate gray.

Amygdaliform (spores): almond-shaped.

Amyloid: referring to spores that become bluish-gray in contact with iodine reactive.

Anastomosed: thickly intervening lamellae, or joined together

Ring: residual of partial veil, that is of a more or less consistent membrane, which, of the young carpophar, joins the margin of the cap to the stem of some species of Agaricales, and then tears and falls back on the stem, encircling it.

Annex: referring to the lamella that reaches the stem and, therefore, can be both adnated and decurrent.

Apical: located at the top, at the apex of the stem.

Appianato (hat): spread out, flattened.

Appendicolato: it is said of a flaky fringe formed by velar residues protruding from the edge of the hat. If referring to the stem, it indicates that it has a thinned, rooting or taproot base.

Appressate: it is said of very narrow gills, approached, precisely appressate.

Areaoso: similar to a spider's web.

Arched: cut of the gills clearly concave.

Areolate: cracked, broken in areoles, that is, in geometric mosaic designs, in tesserae, often due to drought.

Armilla: ring, bracelet, typical of some Basidiomycetes in which there is a single (general) veil that wraps the whole cap and part of the stem and, tearing itself, leaves on the upper part of the latter a sort of collar.

sac, microscopic organ that contains the spores of Ascomycetes.

Ascomycetes: fungi characterized by the ascus in which the spores are formed.

Attenuated: thinned.

Base: lower part of the stem.

Basidium: microscopic cell from which the spores in Basidiomycetes are externally produced.

Basidiomycetes: fungi whose spores are produced on the outside of the basidia

Bifurcate: gills that split near the stem or the edge of the cap

Bulb: swelling at the base of the stem in the shape of a tuber or onion, more or less rooting. stem with bulb at the foot.

Caduco: not very resistant.

Campanulate (cap): bell-shaped, parabolic.

Canaliculate: (stem) with fairly deep parallel depressions, similar to canals.

Cappelloopileus: upper part of the carpophore.

Flesh: internal pseudotissue or pulp of the carpophore.

Fleshy: it is said of the flesh of the stem or of the cap that breaks easily without showing a fibrous-resistant texture.

Carpophor: fruiting body of the upper fungi that is home to the reproductive organs ascus and basidia), improperly called fungus or mycete

Cartilage: consistent and elastic like cartilage tissue

Casing: chalky flesh

Caulocystidia: cystidia placed on the surface of the stem

Cavernous: with small irregular cavities in triples, like caverns.

Cable: empty.

Cercine: ring superimposed on others, formed by velar residues.

Cespitoso: attached to the base of other specimens, in clumps.

Cheilocystidium: sterile cell of the hymenium arranged on the edge of the lamellae.

Cyanophilic: referred to cell wall which turns blue in contact with reagents such as blue-cotton.

Cyliate: with eyelashes, hairs.

Cingulate (ring): toothed wheel.

Cystidium: sterile cell of different shape and function.

Citriform: lemon shaped

Clavate (stem): with club-shaped swelling

Columella: sterile column that starts from the base of the gleba of the Gasteromycetes and insinuates itself into it

Color (of the carpophore or part of it): one of the important macroscopic characters many for the identification of the species.

Connato: born together with other carpophores, bushy.

Color: of the same color.

Convex: it is said to have a hemispherical cap, but with a not very accentuated curvature.

Coverrofile: which likes to grow on the excrements of animals.

Coralid: coral-shaped, that is branched like a coral.

Cortina: partial veil similar to a cobweb.

Corticato: it is said of a stalk that has the external part of the flesh more compact than the internal one.

Crenulate: slightly indented, slightly and irregularly serrated.

Cuticle: film that covers the cap of the mushrooms; sometimes it detaches, it is easily removed from the underlying flesh. So, we talk about a separable cuticle. When it is not possible to detach it, it is an adnated cuticle.

Decurrent (lamella): which runs along the stem.

Deliquescent: fabric that does not rot, but dissolves in a sort of black liquid

Depressed: cap with central depression.

Disc: upper area of the cap more or less central.

Dissociated: (cuticle) broken into more or less regular fragments

Eccentric: not exactly central, generally referred to the stem

Echinulate: decorated with pointed warts

Ellipsoid: ellipse-shaped

Endoperidium: internal membrane of the peridium, located at contact with the gleba.

Epigeo: carpophore that grows on the surface of the soil.

Exoperidium: external membrane of the peridium.

Farinaceous: odor similar to that of flour.

Farinosa: it is said to have a surface covered with a light dust, like flour

Felt: it is said surface covered with fine intertwined hairs

Festonato: fringed hem, wavy

Fibers: small adnate fibers, thin like hair, which line the surface of the carpophore, the cap or the stem of some mushrooms.

Fibrous: covered with fibrils

Fibrous: it is said of flesh which, instead of breaking easily, tends to tear and split according to a fibro-filamentous weave

Thread: cut or edge of the lamellae

Fimicle: coprophil, which loves, develops, grows on the dung.

Fioccoso: sprinkled with flakes similar to those of cotton

Fistulous: crossed by channel. A stem is said to be fistulous, which has a thin canal at its center.

Flabelliform: fan-shaped.

Fugacious: an organ that disappears with age (veil).

Fungal: it is said of the smell of a mushroom.

Frangiato: decorated with residues similar to fringes.

Furfuraceo: covered by a sort of dandruff.

Fusiform: spindle-shaped

Stem: the part of the carpophore that supports the cap or hymenium in general

Gelatinous: as if covered with jelly

Chalky: it is said of a flesh that behaves like gypsum when fractured, a characteristic of species belonging to the genera RussulaeLactarius.

Gibbous: provided with more or less showy protuberances and similar to small humps.

Glabro: naked, without hairs or other ornamentations, but not properly smooth.

Gleba: internal (fertile) part of the peridium of the Gasteromycetes.

Glutinous: covered by gluten, very viscous

Gregarious: associated with other specimens, but not connected

Guttulate: (spore) containing droplets of oil

Habitat: the place, the environment in which an organism develops and, therefore, also of growth of a specific fungal species

Hyaline: transparent and colorless

Ifa: structural unit, threadlike, which, when intertwined with others, forms the mycelium or the web of the carpophore

Hygrophorus: carpophore capable of retaining water, therefore led to turn pale with dehydration and darkening with humidity. Funnel-shaped: it is said of a funnel-shaped cap

Imbricato: caps or scales arranged one on top of the other, like roof tiles

Imenioimenophore: part of the carpophore responsible for reproduction, therefore, containing the basidia and the ascus. referring to the ring): ascending or facing upwards. The opposite of supero.

Inborn: it is said of non-removable ornamentation.

Involute: it is said of the edge of the cap rolled up on itself, facing the i-menophore.

Hypogeum: underground.

Irsuto: covered with spiky hair.

Labyrinth-shaped: tortuous, with an irregular pattern

Lacky: cavernous, it is said of a fabric or surface that, when dissected, has large gaps or cavities inside it.

Lamella: structure similar to a knife blade, arranged with the others in a radial pattern under the cap and on the surface of which are the basidia and, therefore, the sporal dust of the Agaricaceae are housed.

Lamellula: structure similar to the lamella, but shorter, shorter so that it never reaches the stem. Fluffy: covered with soft down, similar to wool: whey emitted by the gills or from the flesh mostly of a Lactarius cut: it can be white, similar to milk or watery, colored, unchanging or turning, acrid or mild

Free: it is said of a gill not attached to the stem. wood.

Lobed: equipped with lobes, that is, with small protuberances.

Spotted: dotted with spots

Marbled: variegated, streaked or veined.

Marginate: it is said to have an enlarged base of the stem, with a shape, that is, a ruined cone.

Margine: peripheral area of the cap, rim, edge.

Membranacea: it is said of a thin structure like a membrane and more or less tenacious.

Mensoliform : (sessile carpophores) that protrude in a shelf from a vertical substrate.

Mycelium: vegetative part of the fungus, formed by an interweaving of hyphae which, among other things, produce the carpophore.

Mycology: science that studies fungi.

Mycorrhia: symbiosis between fungi and roots of higher green plants.

Micron: microscopic unit of measurement corresponding to 1/1000 of 1mm.

Miter: apical part, similar to a bishop's miter, represented by the cap of some Ascomycetes Mucillaginous: covered with semifluid-gelatinous mucus

Naked: it is said to have a smooth cap or stem, that is, devoid of any form of ornamentation. with minute and deep central depression in the shape of a navel.

Hem: margin.

Papillate: equipped with papilla, small well-defined umbo.

Parabolic: in the shape of a parabola.

Parasite: individual who lives behind other living organisms damaging them.

Peridium: outer layer that envelops the gleba of the Gasteromycetes.

Peristoma: small conical crater located at the apex of the ostiole.

Pigment: substance present in the hyphae that gives color.

Pore: orifice, terminal part of a tubule of a boleto or of a polyporus.

Practice: growing on the lawn.

Pruinato: dusted with bloom, a sort of removable powder, formed by aggregates of cells, usually white.

Powdered. Pubescent: with short and soft hair.

Pulvinated (referring to the hat): in the shape of a pillow.

Radicating: it is said of the base of a stem that sinks into the ground like a root.

Tapered: attenuated.

Resupinate: adherent carpophore completely to the substrate with the dorsal part.

Reticulated: decorated with a lattice.

Reticulum: a sort of imprint left by the pores on the stem.

Revivescence: ability of some dried carpophores to resume their primary appearance following rehydration.

Revolved: facing, crumpled outwards, generally referred to the edge of the hat.

Rimoso: equipped with a dense series of fibrils that leads to cracking and therefore to glimpse the underlying tissues.

Rhizomorphic: mycelial formation organized in long bundles of hyphae, similar to a root and suitable for the spread of the fungus in the soil.

Sclerotium: compact and hard cluster of hyphae closely united to form corpispheroidal or elongated bodies able to survive for a long time, even in the presence of atmospheric conditions that are not always favorable.

Scrobiculate: marked by scrobicles, i.e. small dimples.

Scrobicule: small dimple.

Silky: similar to a silk cloth, i.e. with a shiny appearance

Textile: without stem

Spherocysts: spherical cells present either on the cuticle of the hat, in the veil or in clusters in the flesh of the Russules

Sinuous: wavy, lithe

Margin: lamella that just before inserting itself on the stem it rises upwards and then falls again immediately afterwards to connect to it

Margin (referred to the stem): enlarged bulb in the shape of an onion, heart, branch or top Spatoliform: shape of the carpophore more or less like a tongue or a spatula.

Spermatic: referred not only to the smell of human sperm, but also to that emanated from cheese rind, from moist flour, from sausages.

Spore: mass deposit of the spores emitted by the fungus.

Spore: element proposed for the reproduction of fungi whose dimensions usually range from 3 to 20 microns.

Squamulous: equipped with minute scales.

Scales: flat scales, made up of hyphae, which decorate the carpophore.

Jamb: stem of the mushroom.

Striated (for transparency): it is said of the cap margin that allows a glimpse of the underlying lelamellas.

Subgleba: part underneath the gleba, usual y with a spongy, sterile consistency.

Substrate: material on which a mycelium lives, feeds and develops.

Taxon: taxonomic category.

Terricolo: that grows in the earth and not on wood.

Tomentose: covered with fine and short hair, but not exactly velvety.

Texture: the pseudotextile that forms the carpophore

Tubercle: small protuberance placed on a surface (usually on the cap or stem)

Tubule: tube inside which the basidia and, therefore, the spores are arranged. It is open to the outside in the pore.

Turbinate: in the shape of a spinning top or onion.

Ubiquitous: growing in any place and on any substrate.

Umbonate: cap with a rather pronounced protuberance in correspondence with the disc.

Umbone: a sort of more or less pronounced rise in the center of the cap.

Uncinato: attached to the stem and running for a short distance.

General veil: veil (thin membrane) that wraps the carpophore in the first stages of growth.

Partial veil: membranous veil with a protective function of the hymenium.

Venous-joint: it is said of a lamella joined to another by transverse ribs; anatomized.

Ventricose: it is said of a pot-bellied stem, swollen in the median area or of lamellabombata.

Verruca: flattened and floury plaque or minute globose, pyramidal or truncated cone-shaped plaque present on the cap, residue of the general or universal veil.

Hairy: hairy, bristling with hair.

Virante: flesh that changes color in contact with oxygen in the air.

Viscous: covered with a layer of gluten.

Volva: residue of the general veil placed at the base of the stem. It generally occurs in the form of a membranous envelope, a sheathing bag.

Xerophile: loving dry soils and climates.

HABITAT AND GROWTH

Favorable conditions. The habitat represents the most favorable environment, more suitable for the development of a fungus, meaning by this term not only a type of soil with a relative type of vegetation, but also the set of all those chemical-physical conditions and more suitable meteorological conditions that characterize a natural environment. The scarce or abundant growth of a fungal species is closely related to an ideal combination of these conditions, an ideal combination that varies from species to species and which means that in different conditions different fungi can form and develop. In general, however, the factors determining an environment favorable to fungal growth are:

- the nature of the organic substrate, which should be rich in sugars, fats, nitrogen compounds, mineral elements, etc;

- acidity of the substrate, with most suitable pH values between 5 and 7;

- the presence of suitable plant species;

- temperature of the substrate and of the surrounding atmosphere, generally hot-humid climate and in any case absolutely not windy.

Territories with a temperate climate are certainly more favorable to the presence of mushrooms. It is enough to remember how the mycelium is almost always sunk into the ground to understand how vegetation affects its temperature.

The soil, on the other hand, absorbs and retains heat the more it is dark in color and rich in humidity, from which it follows that this type of soil is more favorable to fungal development than the light, calcareous one, with scarce reserves of water;

- abundant availability of water for both the vegetative phase and the reproductive phase;

- presence of light, often important for the development of carpophores.

However, it should be emphasized that the absence of any of the conditions described above does not absolutely negate the formation and development of mushrooms, which, as passionate hunters often tell, can however also be found in particularly hostile environments. which these factors combine and influence each other, so it must be assumed that the appearance of "fungi", of any species, is entrusted to the creation of particular thermal, water and insulation conditions, which are combined with a favorable chemical and physical composition of the soil in which the mycelium is found to vegetate, represented by the first 15 cm below the soil level.

In general, it must be assumed that a good birth of "mushrooms" is possible if there has been a long enough period in which the soil has maintained a good degree of humidity and a high enough temperature, above zero, so that the mycelium can expand and be able to provide for the accumulation of nutrients to be transferred then in the carpophore.

Snow-covered winters, rainy and temperate springs, hot and dry summers followed by temperate autumn seasons with abundant rainfall are therefore favorable; but above all, it is necessary that the wind does not take over, which by drying the soil and the humidity present in the air, is the element most opposed to the release of the "mushrooms". In fact, experienced hunters look forward to the rains, especially in late summer and early autumn, followed by beautiful days and temperate nights. The mycelium has a constant need for water to develop.

The carpophore, on the other hand, sometimes begins to form only when the mycelium begins to experience a certain lack of water, as if, "feeling" close to a period of stagnation, it uses the accumulated food reserves, quickly producing the fruit, necessary for the perpetuation of the species. It is obviously very difficult for all the favorable conditions to occur in a timely manner (the French mycologist Georges Becker has pointed out, for example, that truly abundant seasons follow a rhythm of at least ten years) it is therefore up to the seeker to identify the various particular areas that adapt to the conditions set out above.

Thus, for example, it can assume that in the cold and humid seasons the mushrooms appear only n open clearings or in any case in areas exposed to the sun, that if it is hot but the earth and the air are dry, the mushrooms snack in the more humid, shady, north-facing areas. The following is an attempt by a prospector to describe some trends verified in years of research for "porcini" mushrooms:

"In good years, at the start of the harvest season, the first specimens of porcini will undoubtedly be found at lower altitudes."

Like agronomic crops, mushroom fruiting also follows a trend from "bottom" to "top", initially preferring chestnut woods over other types of vegetation. The first collections, generally scarce, limited to a few specimens, can therefore be carried out in the chestnut groves at 400-700 meters above sea level. With a delay of a few days, it will then be possible to find the first specimens in the beechwood belt, at a higher altitude. The beech forest represents the most constant forest vegetation, in the sense that the growth, between ups and downs, continues throughout the season.

At the same time, the birth will affect oak woods, even at low altitudes, in which however the abundance is strictly correlated, more than in other types of vegetation, to an accentuated rainfall. Within the wooded types, it should then be emphasized that mushrooms generally follow a trend from open, sunny areas to more dense areas. The first specimens of mushrooms will be found in the places exposed to the sun, often among the stones.

Only after a few days will they begin to appear next to isolated clumps, including juniper, first outside them and then more and more inside. Subsequently it is the moment of the thickest grass and, finally, of the shadier undergrowth. "It goes without saying then that even in this case only experience, and therefore only assiduous practice, can produce constant and appreciable results." It should be emphasized that the climatic characteristics described above are not perfectly suited to all species of fungi; it is not uncommon, for example, that seasons rich in fungal species of the most diverse do not see the appearance of other perhaps more sought-after species (this is the case, for example, of the "Porcino" which, unlike other species, will hardly appear abundantly in the autumn season following a very humid and rainy summer). As indeed the opposite consideration is not infrequently valid, giving rise to the phenomenon of the so-called "spy fungi", the discovery of which indicates with a certain probability the presence of other certain species (this is the case, for example, of Amanita muscaria compared to with porcini

GROWTH RATES OF MUSHROOMS

How many times have you heard that mushrooms grow in a few hours? or that instead they need several days? or have you even heard someone talk about 20 days! Surely each of you will have been informed and will have come to your own personal conclusion.

To have more certain and precise answers, however, the questions should be asked of a mycologist, or even a biologist, who has thoroughly studied molds and therefore fungi, including the growth rates from the development of the mycelium to the birth of the carpophore or fruiting body. .

In twenty years of research both from my experience in the field and for having heard many people, including expert mycologists, I have learned a lot. Furthermore, in all these years I have been able to keep an eye on various species of mushrooms, so, taking data on paper, I was able to realize, on the basis of certain facts, how much more or less it takes a mushroom to grow. Obviously we are talking about relative and not absolute data.

However, each mushroom has different growth rates from the others and is dependent on climatic factors.

However, it must be borne in mind that there are many factors that can affect growth and that, if each of these factors is not found at the appropriate level, it can become limiting and

[98]

therefore cause a slowdown in growth, or even a temporary or total arrest.

Below I will list the main and most important factors for the growth of each type of edible fungus:

- the water

- the air temperature

- the soil temperature

- the humidity of the air

- the wind

- the light

- the type of soil

As even one of these factors varies, the growth rate increases, decreases or stops. Think of the arrival of cold wind, the scarcity of water in the ground, a sudden drop in temperature.

Let's take the porcini   as an example

To facilitate understanding and not to go too far, I will take the boletus as an example, because obviously every mushroom, as I said before, has different growth rates from other mushrooms. Having the opportunity, I was able to follow, several times, the growth of various mushrooms, both in the mountains and in the hills, and I noticed that the development in the mountains is slower than in the hills. This is mainly due to the temperatures. In the mountains, night temperatures are often low, even if they reach 25 degrees during the day. It often happens that after strong afternoon thunderstorms the temperature drops sharply and that at night it can even reach 2-3 degrees. In those hours when the temperature is not optimal for the development of the porcini the latter stops its growth.

In the hills, however, the temperature range is less. In general, if the temperature, air humidity and soil humidity are at optimal levels and the wind is almost absent in the hills, the boletus needs about 4-5 days to grow from 1 cm. to dimensions of 10-15 cm. In the mountains, however, the times are longer and vary from 10 to 15 days to get to the same size! It is therefore easy to understand the reason for these differences between mountains and hills.

It is therefore wrong to believe in the almost instantaneous growth of porcini! And this is denied, not only by me, but by any biology or mycology book. Another period to take into consideration is that of the development of new mycelium. When it hasn't rained for many weeks and therefore the soil is dry, the mycelium of porcini, like that of other mushrooms, needs a few days to form new mycelium which will then give life to new fruiting bodies. This is why, usually, after a long drought even if it rains a lot, no mushrooms are seen in the woods before at least 10-14 days pass!! Give it a try yourself. In September, keep an eye on a dry forest and as soon as a moderate rain arrives, try to go looking for mushrooms several times over a 12–14-day period.

You will find that even if the climatic conditions are ideal for the growth of any fungus you will not find mycetes until the 10th or 11th day that goes well and always that unfavorable factors do not intervene to slow down the growth even more. Next time I will talk to you in more detail about my data collected over various years and the growth rates of the various types of porcini (Boletus edulis, Aerus, reticolatus..).

GROWING FRESH MUSHROOMS AT HOME: A PRACTICAL GUIDE

Gathering them in the woods is wonderful, but knowing how to grow mushrooms at home, seeing them grow and enjoying them as soon as they are ready at any time of the year is an even more satisfying experience. Let's see together the simplest techniques for growing fresh mushrooms even in small domestic spaces. Why buy them at the supermarket at often prohibitive prices when you could learn how to grow fresh mushrooms directly in your home in a simple and cheap way? The direct cultivation of mushrooms is the best alternative to harvesting in the woods (linked, moreover, to the seasonality of the product as well as the possibility of dedicating oneself to research) and to buying from the greengrocer. Through our suggestions you will discover how to grow fresh mushrooms and obtain generous harvests free of chemical or phytosanitary residues.

[101]

If you want to know how to grow good and good-looking mushrooms in every season of the year, just follow some practical advice and learn the basic techniques that we will show you in this simple guide dedicated to the direct (and home) cultivation of some of the most common edible mushrooms, such as champignons, oysters and shiitakes, but once you have mastered the technique you can try your hand at growing many other species of fresh mushrooms.

How to grow mushrooms

What do we need?

- ✓ 1 box of wood, plastic or polystyrene with high edges
- ✓ 1 substrate suitable for the growth of mycelia
- ✓ 1 plastic sheet
- ✓ 1 good garden soil
- ✓ 30 gr of ready-made champignon mycelium
- ✓ dry leaves or straw

GROWING MUSHROOMS IN BOXES IS SIMPLE, EVEN FOR THE LESS EXPERIENCED

Preparation. The direct cultivation of mushrooms in the home generally takes place in boxes (made of wood, plastic or polystyrene). On the market you can buy ready-to-use boxes complete with guides on how to grow mushrooms, otherwise you can easily set up your mushroom farm using the common boxes for fruit and vegetables.

The substrate should be a mixture of well-seasoned manure, straw and dry seasonal residues. Also, in this case it is advisable to contact a nurseryman, an agricultural shop or a farm directly. The soil to be mixed must be not too acidic and well sterilized: first pass it in the oven at 80 ° C and store it in a closed bag in the dark until use.

To successfully cultivate your mushrooms, the correct preparation of the mushroom bed is very important: the plastic sheet, possibly dark in color, must be positioned on the bottom of the box in order to cover the entire interior. Use pegs to secure it to the cassette and let it protrude from the sides to fold it back to cover the substrate when ready.

The mixture of manure and soil must be mixed very well and enriched with materials that give softness and porosity to the substrate, such as leaves and straw. In any case, by purchasing the ready-made compound, you will not need to resort to other materials.

The cassette should be filled up to 5cm from the edge, moistened and left to rest for a couple of weeks before use. After this period, you can proceed to burying the mycelium by making small holes in the substrate at a depth of 3-4 cm, 10-12 cm away from each other. Once covered with other substrate and wet with water, the ambient temperature must never drop below 20 ° C. Watering must be daily, avoiding excesses and water stagnation.

The ideal place to grow fresh mushrooms indoors is a garage, cellar, basement or an outdoor place sheltered from the sun and wind. A balcony, terrace, garden, simple window sill or even an enclosed space is fine as long as it is under certain temperature / humidity conditions.

To obtain generous yields, the ideal is to grow champignons with the box technique

The only drawback of growing mushrooms at home is related to the smell of mold that could be generated by the substrate of the mycelium. To grow mushrooms quickly and lastingly, in fact, the perfect temperature is 25 °, anyway, between 20 and 30 °. After two or three weeks from the burial of the mycelium you will see a whitish mold appear, the most evident manifestation of the fungus that begins to grow. Cover it with a thin layer of smoothed, compacted and moistened limestone and use the edges of the plastic sheet to cover the box. In this phase the mushroom farm must be transferred to a decidedly colder environment (12-14 °) keeping the watering constant. After 15-20 days you will see the first mushrooms appear which from tiny will quickly become quite large and full-bodied.

HOW TO GROW MUSHROOMS WITH WOODEN LOGS

If you do not have much time or familiarity with do-it-yourself and you want, know that there are ready-to-use kits on the market (the tee pee kit) that will allow you to grow mushrooms of different varieties and types in a really simple and immediate way. These are pre-inoculated strains with mycelium spores that can also be purchased online on specialized sites such as fieldforest.net where you can also find many practical tips on how to grow mushrooms all year round without ever leaving home.

Mushroom cultivation using a wooden log

In this case you will need:

- ✓ 1 large container and a box to wet and keep the log moist
- ✓ 1 plate just wider than the log
- ✓ 1 spray bottle
- ✓ fresh water without chlorine

Preparation. Place the stump in a shaded area, possibly outside, water it regularly and be patient for at least six months. During this period the mycelia will slowly develop inside the stump until you see the first fruits emerge from the holes. This technique is perfect for growing shiitake mushrooms, a highly regarded variety of Japanese mushrooms and the second most consumed mushroom in the world.

HOW TO GROW MUSHROOMS WITH TOILET PAPER

If you love to experiment with unique (not to say bizarre) cultivation techniques, one that is quite known for growing mushrooms at home is the one based on the use of toilet paper rolls. In this way you can grow edible mushrooms of the oyster variety, which are particularly meaty and tasty. To do this you will need:

- ✓ 1 roll of toilet paper
- ✓ 1 tee pee kit (or buy separately spores, plastic bags with filters and rubber bands)
- ✓ 1 box
- ✓ 1 large, round plate
- ✓ 1 sprayer
- ✓ fresh water without chlorine

Preparation. Fill a pot with water and bring to the boil. Meanwhile, remove the cardboard tube from your toilet paper roll and immerse it in boiling water with the heat off. When it is well soaked, let it drain and cool, taking care not to break it.

Oyster mushrooms grow rapidly in toilet paper rolls

When it is still warm, put the roll in the plastic bag contained in the kit and fill it with the grains containing the spores. Close with the special rubber bands and place the bag on a round plate and place it in the box. Place the box in the dark, in a fairly humid environment and within 3 weeks you will begin to see the first fruits grow.

At this point, place the bag in the refrigerator for 48 hours: the low temperature will accelerate the development of the mushrooms and will allow you to anticipate harvest times. After a couple of days, take the bag from the fridge and remove the roll, letting it rest at room temperature and in a lighted place for a few more days. Regularly moisten the roll with the sprayer.

After 7-10 days the mushrooms will be ready and once removed from the roll (without using knives) just close the bag and wait for the mycelium to reappear to repeat the operation from the beginning.

As soon as you become familiar with one of these three techniques, you will discover that learning how to grow mushrooms at home is really simple and fun, as well as rewarding. You can share this activity with your children and cultivate that little dream of self-producing food that you have been nursing for a long time.

HOW TO GROW MUSHROOMS AT HOME: OTHER HOME KITS AND ORIGINAL SYSTEMS

As we said, on the market we also find a series of more or less effective kits or systems that allow you to try your hand at home cultivation of mushrooms, as well as many other varieties of vegetables and aromatic herbs.

There is no shortage of particularly creative systems, such as the one devised by the Danish designer Jonas Edvard who has created an extravagant biodegradable lamp designed precisely for growing mushrooms at home without the need for soil, boxes, coffee grounds or organic material.

Thanks to the vegetable fibers of which it is composed and to the mycelium (the vegetative part that favors the spontaneous growth of mushrooms), in fact, Myx is able to stimulate the growth of a good quantity of mushrooms (500-600 gr) in just 2 weeks, and directly on the surface of the lamp. During this time, the mushrooms eat the soft plant tissue and thrive on the topmost part of the lining throughout the vegetative cycle.

The mushrooms thus obtained, of the genus Pleurotus Ostreatus, are edible and after harvesting, the biodegradable fabric of the lamp can be composted or thrown away. If used for composting, the waste material will be particularly rich in nutrients thanks to the reproductive and vegetative activity activated by the mushrooms during their growth.

HOW TO GROW MUSHROOMS ON WOODEN LOGS WITH FRESH MYCELIUM

To grow mushrooms on wooden logs with Fresh Mycelium, you must have freshly cut logs avai able, no more than 7/10 days, with an ideal diameter (for a good arrangement) of about 25/30 CM, and 70 - 80 cm long, cut the trunk into slices of 10/15 CM, the first slice is a good idea to make it 30 / 40CM so that you can bury a little in the ground after the trunk has been cloned, when we will then plant it.

The ideal is to make logs of up to 3 or 4 slices including the largest initial slice, so as not to have them bulky for arrangement.

1ST PHASE

Before putting the mycelium on the slices, take 2 or 3 nails and nail them to the ends of the slice by dividing them, and nailing a few centimeters, and leaving half part on the surface, then cut the head of the nail at 45 ° put the mycelium on the slice, and the slice that comes above the nail slcwly, until it is absent with the mycelium, having done this, the slice is nailed and would not move for the arrangement. Obviously get quality nails, new and made of stainless steel. If you do not want to use this method, go to the place where you put them to incubate so as not to move them after having done the appropriate operations.

2ND PHASE

The finished trunks must be closed in plastic bags, such as those of the garbage, it is important that they are clean and new, it is a good idea, however, to let everything breathe, then seal without letting animals enter, and insert at the edge of the bag before closing it, some filters to breathe, even the yellow sponges like upholstery of the chairs are fine. Once this is done, they will then be incubated in a sheltered place at 20-25 ° C, for 2/3 months depending on the variety you choose to grow.

3RD AND LAST PHASE

After the incubation period according to the variety criteria, if you see the trunks covered with a visible layer of mycelium, the plastic bag can be removed, and they can be placed in the garden buried a little, but always sheltered from direct sun and wind, or put them in containers with earth and place them in a corner of the garage, cellar, etc., it is important that the soil remains moist, but avoid stagnant water, where they will then produce mushrooms several times both in Spring and in Autumn.

Well, if everything is done correctly, you are ready to just wait for the mushrooms.

Depending on the variety of mushroom, but some woods that can be used, are:

Poplar, Birch, Willow, Maple, Elm, Linden, Alder, Beech, Walnut etc ...

The best results for different varieties are obviously obtained on Poplar logs

SUBSTRATE FOR MUSHROOMS

In this chapter we will talk about a topic that is generating a growing interest: the substrate for mushrooms.

The substrate is a particular preparation that is found inside the bales of mushrooms to allow their cultivation right at home.

Introduction to Mushroom Substrate

People's awareness of wholesome foods has grown. In fact, many are paying greater attention to the consumption of healthier foods which is at the same time very rich in substances and nutrients that are very important for our health.

The cultivation of some species of mushrooms at home allows us to control day by day the growth of this little used food, however very precious for our body.

This means that more attention must be paid to natural foods, even if not well known, but which contain vitamins, proteins, mineral salts and other important elements necessary for the well-being of our body.

In the cultivation of mushrooms at an amateur level, no special tools or spaces are needed: a cellar, a garage, a garden or even just a terrace is enough to try out this activity.

The satisfaction that will be obtained from it will be great and will also be rewarded by the benefits that mushrooms will do to our body.

Benefits of growing mushroom with substrate

The supply of mineral elements and a natural diet with a higher intake of vegetables and vegetables help us to live better.

The mushrooms grown with the inoculated substrate allow us to have a controlled food, therefore it's certainly healthy.

Here are some important properties that mushrooms have:

- ✓ they contain very few sugars and fats so they are indicated in diets;
- ✓ they are rich in minerals such as phosphorus, magnesium, potassium, selenium, copper, calcium and other antioxidant substances that stimulate and strengthen the immune system;
- ✓ they fight free radicals and therefore slow down the aging of skin and bones;
- ✓ they contain numerous vitamins, including vitamins of group B, group C, vitamin D and others;
- ✓ they contain amino acids and proteins, so they are also useful in vegetarian and vegan diets;
- ✓ they are generally cholesterol-free.

These are just some of the basic properties of mushrooms grown with the mushroom substrate, others are more specific depending on the species chosen.

We can have all this comfortably at home, growing some species with the substrate for mushrooms and monitoring their beginning and development step by step.

The solution? Purchase the bales with mushroom substrate. On the market, there are special kits, if you want to try your hand at this type of cultivation. They are real packages that, in different forms, contain the substrate "seeded" with the spores and the mycelium. Thin filaments, consisting of hyphae, which make up the vegetative part of the fungus. Typically located in the substrate (wood, soil, dung etc) ...

For example, if you want to grow pleurotus mushrooms at home you can order this special kit.

MUSHROOM SUBSTRATE: WHAT SPECIES CAN BE GROWN?

The species of mushrooms that can be grown are different.

Of course, each species of mushroom needs a suitable substrate to recreate as much as possible the natural environment on which it grows, even if the treatments to promote fruiting are similar for all, with particular attention to the temperature compared to the cultivation period.

These are the cultivable mushroom species that need little care and that ensure a more than satisfactory success.

Substrate Pleurotus mushrooms

The substrate for Pleurotus consists of organic material based on various types of straw and other organic components.

Substrate for Champignon Mushrooms

It is one of the most common mushrooms used for growing at home.

The substrate of this mushroom species consists mainly of straw of different types and other organic material suitable for the seeding of the spores of this mushroom.

Substrate sale of Champignon mushrooms

This particular type of substrate is the nutrient medium where the fungus develops and lives can be found packaged in bales of mushrooms. These products can be purchased in specialized farms even if, compared to pleurotus bales, for example, it is quite difficult to find.

Pioppini mushroom substrate

This mushroom is one of the best known and sought after for its goodness and is commonly used in many recipes. The poplar mushroom substrate reflects the natural environment on which mainly poplar wood residues or other suitable types of fruit bear fruit.

Cardoncelli mushroom substrate

The substrate for Cardoncelli mushrooms, that is the Pleurotus eringyi, is mainly made up of various types of straw suitably pasteurized to sanitize it.

Substrate for porcini mushrooms

The substrate for porcini mushrooms does not exist.

Although experiments have been made to reproduce porcini mushrooms, this is not possible for a few simple reasons:

- ✓ the genus Boletus to which Porcini mushrooms belong, is not saprophytic, which lives on decaying organic substances, but is a symbiont organism that has a relationship with other living organisms: they both benefit from each other, that is, it needs to associate with plants with which to live in association, contributing to each other's development;
- ✓ the attempts at reproduction that have been made have not brought satisfactory results because the reproduced species are the poorest ones;
- ✓ cultivation times with porcini mushrooms substrate would be too long and therefore not convenient.

However, it is good to reiterate that the mycelium is thin filaments, consisting of hyphae, which constitute the vegetative part of the fungus. Generally located in the substrate (wood, soil, dung, etc.) of Porcini, it does not exist on the market.

MUSHROOM SUBSTRATE FOR SALE

On supermarket shelves, we can find almost all the mushrooms mentioned above already packaged and ready to be bought. However, growing them indoors is rewarding and will be a source of great satisfaction.

Lately, with the increase in demand for this product, many companies specialized in this sector are emerging.

Studies and trials are therefore being conducted to provide mushroom substrates with a high guarantee of success.

The simplest, most practical and fastest way to obtain this type of product is to order the mushroom substrate packed in mushroom bales, directly from home online, without wasting time looking for specialized dealers that are not always easy to find.

For example, you can order from one of our suppliers a kit for pleurotus mushrooms that is very easy to use and produces several kilos of mushrooms in a season.

Substrate for mushrooms price

The price of the mushroom substrate varies according to the species chosen and the size or weight of the bale that contains it.

They can range from 20 euros to 60 euros and up.

There are kits that include more bales with Read substrate of the same species and, in this case, the prices are more variable.

For example, 4 pieces of bales with substrate for growing Cardoncello can cost 40 euros.

How to grow substrate for fungi

Growing mushrooms with mushroom substrate is not difficult at all, but you have to follow some simple precautions that are provided to those who buy it.

Each species has some characteristics to respect.

It is important to place the substrate, often packaged in bales, in a shady place not exposed to direct sunlight, even better on the terrace or garage or cellar or small greenhouse also to keep it within a certain temperature. The substrate for fungi must be kept moist with regular nebulizations until the formation of the mycelium thin filaments, consisting of hyphae, which constitute the vegetative part of the fungus. Generally located in the substrate (wood, soil, dung, etc.), that is that kind of white mold which, after a few days, will "invade" the substrate.

After a few days, the first fruiting bodies to harvest will begin to appear.

In short, nothing complicated indeed, seeing the substrate bear fruit. It is the nutrient medium where the fungus develops and lives .... Reading about mushrooms will be fun and who knows it could lead to a real passion.

MYCORIZATION

The term mycorrhiza (from the Greek 'mykos' = mushroom and 'rhiza' = root) represents a characteristic case of 'mutualistic symbiosis' between some fungi and the roots of plants: the two living beings are complementary in using resources and exchange with mutual benefit the sugars produced by the plant and the nutritional elements absorbed more efficiently by the fungus.

Mycorization improves the ability of plants to assimilate nutrients: the main function of fungi is to transport nutrients, making them available for absorption by the roots. The third element that takes part in the mineral assimilation cycle is represented by bacteria, responsible for the primary decomposition of nutrients into simpler compounds (mineral salts).

The contact area between the soil and the root system is called the 'rhizosphere' and is classically divided into three zones:

- ✓ the endorizosphere which extends from the surface of the roots to the first internal cell layers;
- ✓ the rhizoplane, that is the external surface of the roots and the portion of soil where the absorption of nutrients takes place;

✓ the hectorizosphere which consists of the volume of soil in immediate contact with the roots and which can vary in size depending on the type of plant and its interactions with the microbial components of the soil.

Analyzing one cubic meter of good agricultural land it is possible to observe a percentage of organic substance equal to 25% (by weight), of which more than 15% is represented by endomycorrhizal fungi and 5% is constituted by bacteria (in the literature we find concentrations of bacteria equal to 10 million / gram of medium). The soil bacteria are made up of a very large population: they are able to adapt to any substance to be metabolized through the formation of specific groups; their ability allows the system to be highly adaptable to any stress.

Mycorrhiza is the most common type of symbiosis in nature: more than 90% of plant species in natural conditions are mycorrhized. To date, in highly anthropized environments (fields cultivated with chemical fertilizers and urban green), mycorrhizae are often absent or present in a very reduced form, most likely due to the chemical pollution of the soil.

The root system of vascular plants consists of roots of different order, in relation to the age of the root. Only the youngest part, younger than one year, is able to assimilate nutrients from the soil. The mycorrhization contributes to the increase of the assimilation of the plant through the formation of a hyphal intertwining that includes or covers the oldest parts of the roots (no longer active) by transporting the compounds inside them. The fungi in this mutualistic association with the root

[120]

system obtain a constant flow of carbonaceous substrates from the plant. Moreover, this loss of carbon is easily replaced by the plant through the greater speed of the photosynthesis process, an advantage still given to it by the symbiosis with fungal associations. The mycorrhized root is recognized by the absence of root hairs.

The fusion between mycelium and root can take place in different ways:

The ectomycorrhizae: the fungus forms a mantle of filaments (hyphae) around the root and penetrates between the cortical cells forming a reticulum (called 'Hartig') without entering inside of the cells themselves.

The endomicorrhiza: the spores found in the soil germinate in the presence of host roots due to the effect of root exudates. They develop until they reach the root itself, and colonize it by penetrating both through the intercellular spaces and directly into the cells.

The fungus thus spreads through the cortical cells where it branches out forming particular structures (shrubs), responsible for nutritional exchanges with the host plant: the plant transfers the excess carbohydrates produced through photosynthesis, the fungus in turn releases the mineral salts absorbed by the surrounding soil.

The shrubs have a short life: after a few days they degenerate. The considerable development of extramatrical hyphae in the soil allows to explore a considerably greater volume of soil than the single root can do, even far from the root absorption zone, significantly increasing the amount of nutrients that can be reached.

The mycorrhizae are able to solubilize and therefore absorb the organic or mineral forms present in the soil in insoluble compounds, and therefore not directly usable by plants. The greatest absorption of mineral salts from the soil

CULTIVATION OF MUSHROOMS: OPTIMAL TEMPERATURE AND HUMIDITY

The substrate is a live, active product, and as such subject to both animal and vegetable pollution throughout the production cycle, in particular in the incubation phase. The smell emanating from the mycelium during incubation can attract insects and other parasites that can cause damage to both the mycelium and fungi. Therefore, it is recommended the maximum cleaning of all environments both before and during cultivation.

THE CULTIVATION OF PLEUROTUS

Before the arrival of the substrate, it is necessary to thoroughly wash and carefully disinfect the production areas and the surroundings. Upon arrival of the substrate, it is important to unload and arrange the blocks in the shortest possible time; according to the season and the temperature (to avoid overheating in hot periods and bad incubations in cold periods)

It is necessary to record daily the values of the fundamental parameters of the cultivation and therefore: ambient and substrate temperature, ambient humidity, ventilation, wetting, treatments and anything else that is considered important. These recordings on a special CULTIVATION SHEET are essential to be able to direct an intervention in the right direction in case of need.

Three stages of cultivation can be distinguished:

incubation, sprouting and production.

During the incubation phase the substrate temperature should be checked daily. This must be included, in the peak period, between 30 ° and 32 ° (a few degrees more only for the Colombinus species). Above 33 ° it will be necessary to intervene to lower the temperature, mainly by exchanging the ambient air in the most favorable hours depending on the season. In the case of low temperatures, the room must be heated.

Other controls during incubation concern the humidity of the environment to prevent the substrate under the holes from drying out - an environmental humidity of 62/65% is required - monitoring for the presence of insects or other parasites in the environment, against which it is possible to intervene with authorized products that inhibit the deposition of the eggs, and the light which is not necessary but not recommended (if possible, keep the environment in the dark).

Although these controls are not usually burdensome, it must never be forgotten that well done incubation is the foundation of good cultivation success.

An incubation performed at a low temperature causes in the best of cases considerable delays and yields lower than expected, with a greater risk of contamination of the substrate.

High incubation temperatures (over 35 °) can cause overheating and death of the mycelium, considerable delays, poor final results both in quality and quantity.

Therefore, a lot of attention is recommended during this very important phase. At the end of the incubation, the substrate must be uniformly invaded by the mycelium and its structure must be compact. The average incubation duration is approximately 15 days.

The germination phase then begins during which there are four fundamental factors that must be regulated and controlled:

temperature, humidity, ventilation and light.

Ideal temperature:

The temperature must be kept constant, as any changes in this phase are very harmful.

Humidity: must be brought to very high values (90/92%). Coarse wetting on the blocks should be avoided.

Ventilation: completely change the ambient air three to five times every hour. To avoid violent blows of air.

Light: it is essential to illuminate the whole crop with a light intensity of at least 200 lux for at least 12 hours a day. The best quality results are obtained in environments illuminated by natural light, while avoiding unshielded sunlight. Pluerotus mushrooms do not arise in the complete absence of light. This fact is exploited to avoid growth under the plastic packaging film of the block, through the use of covering black polyethylene. When the conditions for germination are respected, there is no difference between black plastic and transparent plastic: black plastic is still positive in the event, even accidental, of failure or partial compliance with the ideal environmental values.

When the first mushrooms appear, the production phase begins. At this point it is necessary to:

- Lower the temperature slightly.

    Decrease the humidity to 80/85%. It has been found that in environments with regular and controlled humidity, production benefits in quality and yield, and arrives at the end without too much difficulty: on the contrary, where the humidity is inconstant, the need for wetting the mushrooms frequently causes specific problems. such as bacteriosis, fungal malformations, delays and production losses.

    Gradually increase the ventilation up to 8/10 complete changes of the ambient air every hour.

    Increase the light to the maximum possible, while avoiding direct sunlight and respecting the minimum of 200 lux.

    We underline the often-unrecognized importance of light: in conditions of poor light, mushrooms lengthen the stem, lose color, do not develop normally and can show deformations.

Even if there is a control instrumentation (e.g. thermostats, humidistats, CO2 meters) t is still highly recommended that the grower equip himself with instruments for controlling temperature, humidity and air speed (in order to calculate the actual air changes).

The direct measurement and the immediate association of the measured data to the obtained results can give rise to the repeatability of positive results, and to avoid negative ones.

To conclude, we must never forget that the substrate is an organic product with high humidity and therefore subject to parasitic attacks of various kinds, especially if not kept in good growing conditions.

Mycelium and fungi are very delicate living organisms, comparable to the products of the most specialized agricultural crops and therefore need a lot of care and professionalism.

CHOICE OF SPECIES

Which mushrooms can be grown and which cannot?

Saprophytic fungi and symbiotic fungi

Not all species of mushrooms are suitable for cultivation. To understand which mushrooms can be cultivated we must introduce two main categories of mushrooms: the saprophytic ones and the symbiotic ones. It is much easier to cultivate saprophytic mushrooms because they live on residues of organic substances in a state of decomposition and for these it is enough to recreate the ideal microclimate for their survival and growth. For symbiotic fungi, on the other hand, in addition to identifying the right habitat and the right diet, it is also necessary to recreate the existing relationship with the plant that hosts them.

Fungi are not part of the plant kingdom and are divided into two categories: macromycetes which are those commonly consumed by humans and micromycetes which are not perceptible to the naked eye (such as molds or yeasts). Only for the first category is it possible to speak of cultivation.

These elements with a particular and complex physical structure feed on organic matter which they absorb and then recycle. Fungi are generated by small "spores", from the spores the "hyphae" (small roots also called mycelium) are generated from which, thanks also to a humid and shady climate, the fruiting body called fungus is generated.

The cultivation of mushrooms does not require special skills and not even huge management spaces.

This practice, increasingly widespread, is facilitated by the fact that on the market you can easily find packaged spores of the most commonly consumed mushrooms such as pleurotus mushrooms and champignon mushrooms

Furthermore, the fungus, which cannot be treated like any other plant, needs a particular "substrate" for its survival. The culture substrate is a set of organic and non-organic materials that provide nourishment in the way and in the doses necessary for the fungus.

For example, horse manure (now replaced by a synthetic substrate made up of agricultural chalk, water, droppings and wheat straw) is ideal for the cultivation of champignon mushrooms and the coprinus comatus mushroom, while the cereal straw adapts to the cultivation of pleurotus, stropharia, flammulina and pholiota mushrooms and the wood is the ideal habitat for honey mushrooms, pioppini, pleurotus ostreatus mushrooms and shiitake (or lentinus edodesi.

Wood sawdust, paper, fabric derivatives and cotton by-products are also ideal substrates.

Mushrooms such as strophia ferri or pholiota aegerita can also be reproduced in the home environment, but with costs that would be higher than the hypothetical selling price, these mushrooms therefore remain cultivable as a hobby and not for business or profit purposes.

Shiitake and oyster are also easy mushrooms to grow indoors. For the former it is better to find a stump with the mycelium already inoculated in the wood, for the oyster a simple roll of toilet paper is enough as a natural habitat.

The most common mushroom crops are those of champignons, which account for 80% of national production, and that of pleurots ostratus (orecchietta or gelone) mushrooms which account for the remaining 20%. Minor but still widespread species are the cardoncello, the pioppino and the cornucopia.

The pleurotus and the cardoncello require reproduction in an ideal environment and on a large scale. These plantations are generally electronically controlled for air conditioning and humidification.

The field mushroom remains the most cultivated mushroom because it is more profitable in terms of yield.

GROWING PORCINI MUSHROOMS IS VERY DIFFICULT, WHY?

On the other hand, there are mushrooms whose cultivation is more difficult. Porcini mushrooms, due to their nature, do not adapt so easily to an environment recreated from scratch.

For their birth it is necessary to clone in the best way the lighting, the environment and the humidity and to give life to this species it is ideal to use soil that has already been the "bed" of other porcini mushrooms. The cultivation of porcini mushrooms is very similar to that of truffles, due to the symbiotic relationship that this mushroom establishes with the plant near which it generally grows. But if cultivation is convenient for truffles in economic terms, for porcini mushrooms the risks and costs do not compensate for the low selling prices. Finally, if for the other species there are substrates in bags ready for use, for the porcini mushroom there is still nothing similar.

DIY MUSHROOM CULTIVATION

To create a real "do-it-yourself" mushroom plantation, just take a sack of jute or a small box, soil, manure and some hay. Eventually you can add dry leaves or material that will decay.

Once the mixture has been prepared, it must be placed in the bag or box with a waterproof bottom trying to recreate the ideal humidity situation, that is, with a wet bottom exactly as much as the surface. Then just take the mycelium and spread it on the substrate. Only at the end should it be covered with a light layer of earth. Once it is protected from light, it is sufficient to maintain the optimum humidity level.

HOW TO GROW PLEUROTUS OSTREATUS

the mushroom pleurotus ostreatus was collected from nature and appreciated for a long time and was known by different names: gelone, orecchietta, ostricone, sbrisa, melina. The various terms used indicate some of the characteristics of the mushroom.

Pleurotus is a fleshy and delicate mushroom ranging in color from gray to brown.

Useful tips on the cultivation of Pleurotus Ostreatus.

It is necessary to respect some parameters to cultivate it in an optimal way.

Optimal cultivation period: Autumn, early Winter and Spring, obviously you can grow it all year round.

Temperature: 15 -20 ° C

Relative air humidity: 90% - relative humidity of the substrate 65/75%

Spray the compounds 2/3 times a day in the case of dry environments, vice versa 2 times every 2 days in humid environments

Compounds should never be exposed to direct sun and wind

However, half-light during the day and not in total darkness is essential.

The mushroom reaches maturity 8/10 days after the appearance of the first carpophores (small mushrooms) and it is necessary to increase the humidity of the air up to about 90%, to avoid an excessive lowering of the temperature this operation can be carried out by having a wet sack placed under the tray and proceeding with spraying of nebulized water.

It is clear that in already humid environments they are ideal. For the production it is necessary to keep the bale away from the rays of the sun and the wind, daylight is essential, so do not store in dark rooms.

If many bales are grown in the same room, it is therefore advisable to make many air changes during production. After fruiting has begun, remember to always keep the humidity level high, the mushrooms will come out of the holes already appropriately prepared, it is not advisable to make other holes.

As soon as you see the mushrooms growing it is advisable to wet them from time to time, it is always recommended with nebulizers. You can pick them as soon as the cap gets bigger and the previously curved edge will tend to straighten. The mushrooms must be picked with a slight rotation and not cut at the base, as it is necessary, in order to have another reproduction, to leave the hole free until the straw is seen again.

Production:

The production of mushrooms will last about 15-20 days then do nothing, leave the mixture to rest and do not water until you see the mushrooms reappear again, and repeat as you did for the previous period, there can be from two to four periods in all, depending on the care with which the bale was held.

During production, the mushrooms can produce spores that you can see in the form of white powder, do not be alarmed it is an indicator that the mushrooms have reached their maximum maturity and therefore must be collected and consumed.

The climate:

It is of primary importance for the cultivation of Pleurotus Ostreatus, even if it is called chilblains for its characteristic of bearing fruit even in winter, with temperatures between 4 and 20 ° C.

Too hot sun or too strong wind prevent fruiting in part or in whole.

Drought is a lethal enemy, so the degree of humidity in the growing environment plays a decisive role.

Ambient humidity should be similar to that of autumn days after rains, in the order of about 80/90% with temperatures between 15 and 20 ° C.

These humidity levels are attempted to recreate them in other periods with frequent water sprays on the compound and on the mushrooms themselves.

In cultivation, air circulation is important, which has the function of homogenizing the conditions inside the room in which it is grown, and can be obtained through fans or side openings on the entire perimeter of the room.

The need to change the air satisfies two important conditions:

Removes the carbon dioxide produced by mushrooms, and lowers temperatures where necessary.

While this operation is a little more complicated in winter, as in the presence of cold temperatures outside.

In this case the air exchange must be reduced and partially replaced with a recirculation of the internal air.

In general, the air in the growing environment should be completely changed several times in an hour.

Hygiene:

In mushroom cultivation, prevention is essential.

Before storing the bale, it is necessary to disinfect the premises with products based on quaternary ammonium salts, taking care to have removed any possible organic residue.

These products have a bacterial and sporicidal action at the same time.

It is a good idea to use a larvicidal insecticide as a preventive measure, especially on the walls and ceilings of the premises to prevent possible infestations of midges.

It is essential that the cultivation rooms are easily cleanable and washable, with smooth and non-porous surfaces.

The floor must be as compact as possible and not give rise to water stagnation, preferably covered with a layer of concrete or alternatively with a mulching, filtering, non-slip sheet.

In some cases, hydrated lime is used to spread on the ground, when there is no concrete or protective sheet.

The room must be served by a water network, to carry out the daily watering, it must be located in a protected manner from the prevailing winds, especially if coming from the northern quadrants

PORCINI MUSHROOM

Porcino is the name commonly used to indicate Boletus edulis, an edible mushroom of the Boletaceae family and is the best-known species of the Edules section. The term derives from the Latin edulis and means edible.

The common features of porcini mushrooms have the cap, the upper part of the mushroom, of a velvety brown color, with a size of 10 to 30 cm in diameter and its flesh first has a firm consistency, and is white. It is hemispherical and irregular when young, sometimes not very developed compared to the stem, then flattened, regular and finally convex with raised lobes. The cuticle, which covers the cap, can be thick, thin and separable only in flaps.

It can be smooth or wrinkled but, in wet weather, it is also slimy and shiny. The color varies from light yellow-brown to ocher or white chestnut in youth and turns to greenish or greenish yellow when ripe. The hymenophore is the part located under the cap, it can be lamellar or spongy and serves to contain the spores. It consists of tubules, up to 30 mm long, of soft consistency, easily separable from the cap and of a color first white, then yellowish and finally greenish. The pores are small, round and with tubule colors.

Finally, the stem of porcini mushrooms has the function of bringing out of the ground the structure within which the spores form. It generally has a cylindrical shape, more attenuated at the apex, whitish or light brown in color and dimensions equal to 10 × 15 cm. It has a fusiform structure, more or less fibrous or fleshy but sometimes also elastic and the surface can be smooth, reticulated, velvety or scaly.

HOW, WHERE AND WHEN TO GROW PORCINI MUSHROOMS

In a prized position among the most popular foods of the Italian culinary tradition, ideal for preparing tasty recipes, the porcini mushroom can also be grown and cared for in our garden. The environmental characteristics are fundamental for the growth of porcini mushrooms and cultivation is not easy. It is important to know, in fact, that the fungus lives in symbiosis with the roots of trees, therefore, its cultivation must be organized by recreating the ideal conditions between undergrowth, soil substrate and climatic conditions.

The cultivation of porcini mushrooms starts through the mycorrhization technique which consists in transferring the roots of the fungus to a soil and creating a symbiotic relationship with other higher plants. The ideal trees for cultivating porcini   are mycorrhized oak and chestnut trees - that is, with porcini   spores. They must be in a humid and shady place and with suitable soil.

This last element is fundamental: to attempt a cultivation it is necessary to use a soil in which other porcini have already developed in the past, so that the porcini can receive the nourishment necessary for its growth from the chestnut. The presence of chestnut and beech trees in the area can help cultivation. It is therefore necessary to have a large area characterized by the aforementioned favorable conditions in which to bury the mycorrhized plants and the spores of porcini mushrooms; for which it is preferable to purchase from specialized companies.

Before starting the actual cultivation, however, a soil and climatic analysis is necessary, especially as regards the frequency of precipitation which can compromise the correct evolution of the process.

Since this process is often long and demanding, modern agricultural techniques are experimenting with the cultivation of porcini in greenhouses. It uses the same cardinal principle: the creation of an ideal habitat, in the greenhouse, for the development of a symbiosis between plant and fungus. To achieve this, straw bales are used in which the specially selected porcini mushroom spores are implanted. The spores inside the straw bales require an incubation period between 70 and 90 days, during which regular irrigation must be carried out, morning and evening, and sprayers must also be prepared from above to maintain a humidity. constant. Obviously, this is an experimental technique but the resulting mushroom is very similar to the authentic porcini   in terms of appearance and flavor quality.

What is porcini mycelium

The mother plant from which the porcini mushroom is born is called mycelium, and is an intertwining of filaments or tubules called hyphae. The mycelium can have a long or even very short life and its growth conditions the development of the fungus that constitutes its fruiting body.

To form the mycelium, which is the vegetative body from which porcini mushrooms will arise, it is necessary to meet two primary mycelia of opposite poles. From their union, the secondary mycelium will be born which will develop to produce new fruits, namely porcini mushrooms. The mycelium is also sold on the market in special packages used for the artificial cultivation of the mushroom. To sow the mycelium, it is necessary to dig several holes (depending on the quantity of product purchased) of 30 cm in diameter and 15 cm in depth around the tree.

The holes should be dug at a distance of about 10 cm from the trunk. Then you have to insert the mycelium (1/3 of the pack per hole) and then fill them with earth. Finally, it is important to place a bucket of water around each hole. The mycelium will remain active for 3 - 4 years and porcini mushrooms will start to grow between June and November, the first or second year of sowing.

Varieties of porcini mushrooms

However, there are many different external characteristics, so much so that experts have distinguished at least four species of porcini:

Boletus edulis, commonly known as "bastard, scrub mushroom, September, moccicone";

Boletus aerus or also "bronzino, black mushroom, broom mushroom, moreccio";

Boletus aestivalis, common names "ceppatello, estatino, white mushroom, statoiolo, summer porcini ';

Boletus pinophilus, or also "red head, cold mushroom, porcini of the pines".

The ancient Romans called these mushrooms Suillus for their generally stocky and massive appearance, and the term porcini is the exact translation.

They are generally found in heaths, in oak, chestnut, conifer and beech woods and in high mountain fir forests. These are fungi that can develop in groups of many specimens and easily reach large sizes.

CHAMPIGNON

The champignon belongs to the Agaricaceae family and to the Agaricus genus, that is, rural. Although the term champignon is generic, under this indication we find only edible and good quality mushrooms. Field mushrooms are not classified in the basic food groups because they do not belong to fruit or vegetables. Their nutritional properties are scarce and they have no traces of lactose or gluten. The characteristic of the champignon is the thick and scaly cap of ocher / yellow color. The stem has a more or less stocky ring depending on the species and growth.

WHERE AND WHEN THE FIELD MUSHROOMS GROW

The name suggests the place of growth of mushrooms, which spontaneously arise in meadows. It is important to collect them after having completed the training course or by having them seen by someone competent due to the confusion with toxic and poisonous mushrooms. The growth period goes from spring to autumn and to avoid confusion with other poisonous mushrooms it is good to refer to the color of the gills under the cap. The young champignon has a pinkish lamella gradually turning towards dark brown.

How to grow champignons in a mushroom farm

If the idea is not to go in search of mushrooms in the places or periods indicated, you can choose to cultivate the mushrooms in mushroom farm. First of all it is important to choose a quality compost and it is important to proceed in three stages: a first phase that involves the pre-conditioning and where the raw materials are mixed together and moistened. These will be ready to proceed with the initial decomposition.

Generally, the ideal compost consists of a large amount of manure and straw. The recommended doses are to add 1.5 kg of fat and 1 kg of ammonium sulphate for every 100 kg of straw and manure. If everything is done properly, the compost will overheat and change color within two weeks. The second phase is that of composting, that is, the decomposition is accelerated by rotating the pile every 2-3 days. All with water; just enough to keep it moist. The third and final phase takes place after 2 - 4 weeks. The compost is moved indoors, where the temperature must be kept between 40 and 60 degrees centigrade and will allow the pasteurization process to start. It is important to always monitor the temperature with a thermometer.

Spawning

Spawning is a delicate process that for many producers is not replicable. These in fact buy from a few specialized producers who are able to maintain high standards and guarantee freshness.

Differences between champignons and amanita

The champignon is widely spread and consumed even by those who are not very familiar with the subject. The crux is that this can be confused with an amanita, which is a young specimen of a deadly poisonous angel. In order to differentiate one from the other species it is important to examine the volva or cup at the base of the fungus. If the vault is present then it is amanita. It is necessary to examine the debris, the base of the fungi and the cut of open young specimens to check their gills. In addition, the amanita grows in moss woods and lives in conjunction with the spruce.

Pests and diseases of champignons

Despite the treatments, champignons are not exempt from the attack of diseases and parasites. Prevention is always recommended so that unpleasant unforeseen events do not ruin the entire growth. First of all, it is essential to always work with clean tools and pure equipment and compost. Everything must therefore be uncontaminated by spores. Any sign that may even portend a parasite must be a wake-up call and we must immediately go to the origin of the matter and thus avoid its spread. In fact, it is important to remember that the ideal conditions for the growth of mushrooms go hand in hand with the ideal growth for parasites.

Properties and Benefits

We know that mushrooms strengthen the immune system and fight cholesterol, which is why it is recommended as a food. Both for the few calories it has and for the benefits that these bring to our body. In fact, this food has few calories, is rich in water and low in fat and brings significant benefits to the nervous system and the immune system. They are in fact recommended during the change of season between summer and autumn, combined with a detox diet. The absence of gluten and lactose also makes them accessible to allergy sufferers, except for those sensitive to histamine.

How to cook them

Once the desired result has been obtained in the cultivation of champignons, the long-awaited moment comes to serve them in the kitchen. These, in fact, are a delicious dish if cooked as soon as they are picked. If it is not possible to cook them immediately, the champignon can be wrapped in cling film and left in the fridge for several days. From the ground to the table there are some essential steps that cannot be skipped. First you need to remove the earthy part from the stems with the help of a small knife. Then we move on to cleaning the mushrooms with a damp cloth or through a quick wash under running cold water and subsequent drying. This is the moment when you can choose the dish to use them for. Chopped, fried, thickened. There are various types of cooking, dishes and variations. The mushroom, in fact, unleashes the imagination of all gastronomic lovers.

Varieties of the champignon

The champignon, or agaricus campestris, in addition to being confused with toxic species, can have some varieties within it including: agaricus equestris, floccipes, fuscopilosella, squamulosa or isabelline. A characteristic species is instead the acaricus arvensis; it is a champignon with larger dimensions that reach a good 20 cm in diameter of the cap.

THE AGROCYBE AEGERITA - PIOPPINO

Upon arrival, the bale of Pioppino must have a white mold (even partially) it is the mycelium spores that are inoculating the bale and in doing so create the ideal habitat for the development of the fungus.

1) POSITIONING

The correct position to hold the bale is vertical, in order to have more surface to produce mushrooms. Make small cuts of about 3-4 centimeters (ten is enough) on each side to allow the mushrooms to take air and start growing.

It is important that the block of the bale remains well covered and is sprayed at least once a day.

2) THE PLACE

Ideal for cultivation is humidity, cellars, garages, sheds are preferred, also outdoors making sure that the bale is sheltered from wind and rain.

Not recommended place is at home, especially if heated: dry air does not proliferate, but will regress the fungi.

The birth period is estimated, that s not programmable: sometimes there are bales that produce immediately (probably because they have been sown for some time), other times it is necessary to wait longer because sowing is recent.

The ideal temperatures are from 15 ° to 25 °

3) COLLECTION

The harvest takes place by twisting the mushroom and not cutting it to allow the bale to produce mushrooms again.

4) DURATION OF THE DANCE

Usually, the best time to produce mushrooms at home is from September to November / December. Taking into account that the cold does not help but slows down production, we need to look for a suitable place, like the basement, but with humidity and temperatures that do not fall below 15 °.

The duration of production of the bale from the moment of the first production is about 3-4 months although in some cases it can be up to 6 months after the first harvest. Obviously, the largest collection of mushrooms takes place in the first 2 months, then the production will decrease.

5) HOW MUCH A BALE PRODUCES

A bale of Pioppino produces about 20-30% of its weight, i.e. if the bale weighs 4 kg, the production will be about 1 kg-1.2 kg of mushrooms while for the 13 kg bale the production will be 3-4. kg.

The production estimate is made based on the first 3 months.

6) USE OF THE PIOPPINO IN THE KITCHEN

There are quick and easy recipes to taste Pioppini. In the kitchen they are mainly used to season pasta, from classic risotto to linguine, and tagliatelle.

Also good in a pan with a simple brush of oil and accompanied with chilli, garlic and parsley.

SHIITAKE MUSHROOMS

In nature, mushrooms grow spontaneously during the rainy season. At home, the idea is to simulate the arrival of autumn!

Stimulate fruiting: dip the trunk in cold water. Fill a container with water and keep the log submerged for at least 24 hours.

Remove the watery log and place it vertically on a flat base in a ventilated, warm and humid place, avoiding direct sunlight. The optimum temperature is 25 ° C and humidity 60-70%. If you get these conditions, the productivity of the trunk will be greater.

After 1 to 3 weeks, small white and brown buttons begin to appear in the center (their development will be slower in winter). The mushrooms are ready for harvesting after 3/5 days when the cap is completely open or with the edges slightly curved downwards. If the humidity level in the room is low, it is advisable to spray the logs with water.

Collect the whole mushrooms, without cutting them at the base, but by gently twisting the base of the stem. Mushrooms can be eaten immediately or stored in the refrigerator covered in a food-safe film for up to 2 weeks. If you want, you can also store them frozen or dehydrated: they will retain the flavor and nutritional properties after defrosting or rehydration.

After 2-3 months of each harvest, you can induce new fruiting. Each trunk must not be "stimulated" more than 6 times a year in order not to weaken the germinative capacity of the mycelia of the shiitake mushroom. Between fruiting bodies, "spontaneous" production of fungi can occur due to irrigation. These mushrooms are usually fewer in number but larger.

SPONTANEOUS PRODUCTION OF SHIITAKE MUSHROOMS

As an alternative to the fruit growing scheme, the trunk can simply be left out in the open, laid out on the ground in a shady spot and watered regularly to maintain humidity. Thus mushrooms spontaneously appear, following the rhythm of nature.

FAQ for growers

I opened my Mushi Mini-Log and I already see some dried or rotten mushrooms.

It's natural! Mushi Mini-Log is a living product! In the time between production, packaging and arrival at your home, the trunk may retain some moisture and give life to some small fungus which, not being harvested, will remain there on the trunk. Just remove it and wipe the bark with a damp cloth. In the case of mold (even that is natural and easily removable) you can use a cloth soaked in alcohol.

Where is the best place to grow Shiitake mushrooms with Mushi Mini-log?

Place the trunk in a ventilated, warm and humid place, avoiding exposure to direct sunlight. The optimum temperature is 25 ° C and humidity 60-70%, so the productivity of the trunk will be higher as you approach these conditions. Temperatures below 5 ° C or above 40 ° C can inhibit the growth of fungi and cause the death of the mycelia.

How much should my trunk be watered?

To maintain the right humidity of the trunk it is necessary to carry out periodic watering. The frequency of watering depends on the weather conditions: 1-2 times a week during the summer season; 1-2 times a month during the winter season. To water you can use a sprayer or immerse the trunk directly in water for a few minutes. If the log is too dry (for example if it is lighter than usual or if it begins to crumble in the upper part) it is advisable to keep the log submerged for at least 4-8 hours.

I'm going on vacation, what do I do?

If you will be away from home for more than 2 weeks, place the log in hot water for 1 or 2 days before you leave (this can cause fungus to grow in your absence, but will prevent the log from drying out too much). When you come back, plenty of water.

Few mushrooms have grown from my trunk, what do I do?

The first "production" can be scarce due to the prolonged period of quiescence in which the mycelia are found. Following normal fruit growing cycles, the trunk will tend to produce more fungi. Towards the end of their life cycle, the productivity of the mycelia gradually begins to decrease and the rest time between cycles becomes increasingly greater.

Is there a remedy from the bark sprouting mold?

If mold begins to grow in the bark, reduce watering and place the trunk in a ventilated place: this way the bark stays moist. Mold can be removed by gently brushing the affected area with an alcohol-soaked cloth.

NAMEKO

The Nameko (Pholiota nameko is a small cinnamon-colored mushroom with a slightly gelatinous coating, widely cultivated and consumed in Eastern countries but also in Russia and the United States. Japan is the country that holds a considerable cultivation so that the name nameko derives from Japanese which means slimy mushroom.

In this sheet we will see how to grow nameko, with particular regard to the cultivation substrate and the most suitable environment.

The cultivation techniques of the nameko are very similar to that adopted for another mushroom, namely: the Flammulina velutipes.

The substrate on which to carry out the cultivation of the nameko must consist of broadleaf sawdust. It should be noted that, in some crops, supported by research on the subject, they indicate that sawdust from conifers (Pinus spp. And Cryptomeria japonica) gives better production results.

Rice bran must be added to the sawdust of broad-leaved trees (or conifers) as a supplement; in this case, if you choose coniferous sawdust, the concentration must be 15%, while if you opt for hardwood sawdust, the concentration must be 10%.

Another option, which simulates the natural growth habitat, is to cultivate the nameko with a more natural method,

[154]

using partially buried wooden trunks, in order to guarantee the high level of humidity that the mushroom needs for the growth.

We remind you that for its optimal growth the incubation temperatures must be contained between 24 and 29 ° C, and then lowered to 10-16 ° C to induce the fruiting of the fungus. In this second phase, simultaneously with the thermal shock, the concentration of carbon dioxide (CO_2) must be reduced and the light intensity must be increased, maintaining a high degree of humidity through water nebulisations within the cultivation environment.

Remember that the nameko mycelium is easy to buy even through specialized online sales sites. Alternatively, especially for those who want to try their hand for the first time, there are on the market the mycelium nails which are small wooden cylinders on which the mycelium seed of the Pholiota nameko mushroom has been raised. The cultivation is done on logs of oak, beech, birch, poplar, linden, alder or other broad-leaved trees, but recently cut and therefore fresh and healthy.

STROPHARIA RUGOSOANNULATA

Stropharia rugosoannulata is a baisidiomycete mushroom belonging to the Strophariaceae family.

Systematics

From the systematic point of view it belongs to the Eukaryota Domain, Fungi Kingdom, Basidiomycota Division, Basidiomycetes Class, Agaricales Order, Strophariaceae Family and therefore to the Stropharia Genus and to the S.Rugosoannulata Species.

The terms Psilocybe rugosoannulata (Farl. Ex Murrill) Noordel are synonymous, and Stropharia ferrii Bres.

Etymology

The term Stropharia comes from stróphium, pectoral band, used by girls to tighten the breast: in reference to the ring or its traces often present on the stem of these mushrooms. The specific rugosoannulata epithet derives from wrinkled, rugosus and annulatus with a ring.

Geographic Distribution and Habitat

Stropharia rugosoannulata is a saprotrophic species that grows in the wild or cultivated on soils rich in humus and with vegetable debris, such as fields cultivated with corn, especially with horse manure or in any case on very nitrogenous soil; it is also reported on sandy ground. This mushroom bears fruit especially in spring and more rarely in autumn.

In its spontaneous state it grows gregarious on woody residues of broad-leaved woods, often on sandy soil. It is present in Europe and North America, and also introduced in New Zealand.

Recognition

This mushroom is recognizable as the carpophore can reach dimensions of 15 - 20 cm and more in diameter. The color of the cap can be of various shades, from reddish-brown, red-vinous, violet (yellow in Stropharia rugosoannulata f. Lutea).

The gills are adnate, dense, ash gray, violet with white thread. Cylindrical jamb, attenuated at the base, white, yellowish at the base, often with rhizoid cords, in some cases diffuse and branched, it has a ring with typical streaks.

The stem is tall and is surrounded by a wrinkled ring, hence the origin of the name. The flesh is firm, whitish in color, with a characteristic, almost metallic smell and initially mild and then slightly bitter taste. Under the microscope, ellipsoidal spores, 11-13 × 6-9 µm, smooth, with germinative pore, blackish brown with a purplish brown color can be seen.

Cultivation

Stropharia rugosoannulata is easily cultivable on a substrate similar to that on which it grows in nature. Studies have shown that this mushroom can be grown very well on the same soil as corn. By finding your own preferred conditions, this mushroom can also grow in other types of cultivation, such as medical herbs grown for herbal purposes.

Both the typical form of this mushroom and the lutea form often grow in the same station and at the same time, but without the respective specimens mixing.

Customs and Traditions

Stropharia rugosoannulata, unlike most mushrooms of the genus Stropharia, is an edible mushroom, described as very tasty by many authors, and grown commercially, especially abroad. It is present in the list of marketable mushrooms.

It is grown and marketed abroad, especially the Lutea variety, but its edibility is controversial; in fact, there have been minor gastric disturbances, probably due to collections in polluted places or due to food abuse.

This mushroom, due to the considerable size of the carpophore, is also called "godzilla mushroom".

This mushroom, both for the consistency of its flesh, with its immutable white color, and for its size, immediately found food favor since its discovery. Once it was found to be cultivable on a preferential growth substrate that can be easily reproduced artificially, it has also become a commercially cultivated species in Central and Northern Europe, especially in Germany, Austria and the Netherlands, as well as at an amateur level.

However, in recent years, minor intoxications have been reported, mostly due to gastrointestinal intolerances; it seems that they were caused by specimens grown in the wild, so some authors believe those coming from controlled cultivation are safe. Other authors prefer instead to follow a more cautious line and still advise against consumption.

The large size and the fleshiness of the specimens, together with the color of the gills, allow you to identify this mushroom easily.

The only species that could deceive the less experienced could be the Stropharia hornemannii (Fr.) Also of good size and with similar color especially in young specimens, which however has a stem covered with flaky scales. In the event that the scales are removed, due to excessive manipulation or due to atmospheric conditions, the ring can be observed which in S. hornemannii is fleeting and thin, while in S. rugosoannulata it is broad, persistent and striated above.

Furthermore, young specimens, with closed cap and hymenophore with gills not yet visible, can be so stocky as to resemble a boletus, especially in the case of a cap with a dominant brown color. S. eximia Benedix is also mentioned in the literature, probably due to a completely depigmented form, that is, with a white cap, of S. rugosoannulata.

A 2006 study showed that Stropharia rugosoannulata has the ability to attack the nematode Panagrellus redivivus; the fungus produces spiny cells called acanthocytes which are able to immobilize and digest nematodes.

Preparation Method

This meaty textured mushroom can be consumed, cooked and stored in various ways. To this day there remains the doubt about its certain edibility given cases of mild poisoning which occurred in various parts of the world. One of the reasons could be the presence of unknown material in specimens collected in the wild.

MUSHROOM PLEUROTUS CORNUCOPIAE (GOLDEN MUSHROOM)

Get good quality mold-free wheat straw. Cut it into pieces 2-3 cm long. Water for 1-2 days, stirring so that everything is evenly moist. The mixture will have reached the right degree of humidity when, without spontaneously releasing water but only firmly squeezed between the fingers, it will let out a few drops of water. Get plastic bags of about 5-10 liters. (e.g. bags for storing food in the freezer). Mix the wet mixture with the mycelium (mushroom seed) and fill the bag. Get a piece of clean foam or sponge. Close the mouth of the bag, taking care to place the piece of foam rubber in the center so that the mycelium breathes and develops. Keep the bags with the sown compost at 25-28 ° C for 30-40 days: when everything is invaded by the mycelium, the experiment will be successful and the bag can be taken to the terrace or garden to produce mushrooms! Bring the incubated mixture into the garden, in a corner sheltered from the sun and wind, cut the top of the plastic bag and trim it at the level of the compost, bury it almost completely and cover it with a light layer of earth, keep the earth moist: the first mushrooms will begin to emerge after 15-20 days.

Attention: it is very easy to pollute and affect the final yield. Work the straw in a clean environment with perfectly clean hands. Whenever possible it is good practice to sterilize the processed mixture.

USEFUL INFORMATION

Temperature for the growth of mushrooms: 18-28 ° C.
Quantity of mycelium: 1 jar of dry mycelium of gr. 200 per kg 30
of compost.

COPRINUS COMATUS MUSHROOM (COPRINUS, CHIOMATO AGARIC)

This is well known to all fans for the odd shape of his candle-like cap. it is an appetizing mushroom as long as it is harvested young and consumed quickly.

Get some fresh horse manure (max. 25-30 days) and add about 20% of straw that you have already had the precaution of moistening in a pile for about fifteen days. Wet the mixture perfectly and then form a "mass" of about 1m-1.50m. section and as long as needed: after a few hours the temperature will tend to rise considerably. After four days, undo the "mass" and form small mounds 15-20 cm wide. and 10-15 cm high. and as long as needed: the temperature, measured with a thermometer in the heart of the pile, will tend to rise so much that it will be difficult to keep your hands in the center.

After a further 6/7 days, undo the heap and make it again bringing the external parts inside and vice versa, wet the dry parts and distribute them. The heaps will have to be redone every week until the temperature will no longer tend to rise (once the mass and 3-4 times the heaps). The mixture is now brown, soft, devoid of the unpleasant odor of ammonia and, squeezed tightly between the fingers, it will let out a few drops of water (pH 7.2-7.4). Now is the time to put in the mycelium. Sprinkle the heap of crumbled mycelium (this jar for about 30 kg of mixture thus obtained) then push it in deep with your fingers.

Keep the heap at an internal temperature of 16-20 ° C. After a fortnight, cover it with a thickness of 4-5 cm. of special earth obtained with 4/7 of peat, 2/7 of very small gravel and 1/7 of calcium carbonate well mixed (ph 7.2-7.4). To produce mushrooms in other places, put the mixture in polyethylene crates or bags, press it and cover it with the appropriate earth. Keep the soil well moist and, after about 20-30 days from covering, you will see the first mushrooms appear. After the first harvest while waiting for the following ones, spaced by about 8-10 days between them, the waterings must be sparser.

ARMILLARIA MELLEA MUSHROOM (CHIODINO)

Also known as Chiodino. It grows in groups on freshly cut wood logs with a diameter of about 10-15 cm. Its stem is not edible except for very young specimens, the cap is highly appreciated.

The method, initially conceived on an industrial level, is now only a hobby and it is recommended to implement it using the mycelium (seed) specially designed for logs, as described below.

GENERAL NOTES

Inoculation period: possible all year round but preferably from April to June.

Planting of the inoculated strains: from August to October.

Production: from autumn to spring for 3 consecutive years with expected production of mushrooms amounting to over 20% of the weight of green wood (1/2 in the 1st year, 1/3 in the 2nd year, 1/6 in the 3rd year).

Although it is possible to use the wood of all broad-leaved trees, better results are obtained with poplar.

INCUBATION AND INOCULATION

Use a clean corner of a cool, little used and dark room, eg. cellar.

Spread clean cardboard on the ground, moisten and sprinkle with mycelium (avoid crushing and polluting the mycelium). Arrange a first layer of strains, put other strains, more mycelium and then up to a maximum of 5 layers.

On the last layer distribute more mycelium, cover with cardboard. Cover the mass with well washed jute bags or other clean waste fabrics, moisten and cover again with a polyethylene sheet without sealing.

If everything is regular, we begin to observe the development of the mycelium from the 15th day, at the end of the incubation (2-3 months), the strains are coated with a white patina with a pleasant odor that most of the time also invades the bags of jute, which, in this case, are capable of producing mushrooms.

Warning: the incubation temperature must be kept within 20-28 ° C (if it rises, remove the polyethylene sheet and moisten)

RESIDENCE AND PRODUCTION

Transport the inoculated stumps to the place chosen for production (garden, fields, undergrowth, etc.) and bury them for 3/4 of their height, sheltered from sun and wind.

Keep the stumps that will bear fruit in the period mentioned above moist.

GROWING MUSHROOMS: HOW TO START A PROFITABLE MUSHROOM FARM

In this chapter we will see the various steps, bureaucratic and otherwise, that will guide you in the realization of a successful mushroom growing.

With the crisis of the modern working system, where the permanent job has become a chimera, the need to create a decent job has become essential to live a peaceful and peaceful life.

The contents you see are reported in the most objective way possible because the goal of the blog is to tell the truth without deceiving or encouraging anyone.

However, despite some positive parameters, it should not be forgotten that to start a profitable agricultural business you need a lot of commitment and above all a sales strategy aimed directly at the public.

In fact, one of the first problems for an agricultural entrepreneur is that of marketing. If you can sell to the end customer, the profit margins are such that the business is profitable. Conversely, if you only sell wholesale you will necessarily have to obey the harsh laws of wholesalers that influence prices in an exaggerated way.

An agricultural business is a balanced mix of production, quality, brand visibility and customer confidence. If you have a passion for working in contact with nature, you can find the complete list of dedicated articles in the category "agricultural activities".

The chapter consists of three parts, the first part describes the general situation of mushroom growing, the various cultivable species and the progress of technology, the second part tells in detail how to grow mushrooms for commercial purposes while in the last part we will see how to start a plant successful mushroom cultivation.

A farm has enormous potential for success only if it follows paths such as quality, traceability, environmental sustainability, innovation and promotion.

Mushrooms and mushroom growing

As its name indicates, mushroom farming is the cultivation of edible mushrooms. Mushrooms used for human consumption are part of the "fungi kingdom", a systemic group that is neither part of the animal kingdom nor the vegetable kingdom.

This group contains about 100,000 species, classified for the first time by the mythical Linnaeus, but which in recent years has seen a great reclassification due to new molecular technologies.

Fungi have some characteristics in common that differentiate them from other kingdoms such as strictly heterotrophic nutrition (they cannot synthesize organic molecules from inorganic nutrients), production of spores for reproduction and lack of differentiated tissues.

Fungi play a very important ecological role in nature because they decompose the organic material present in the soil and put it back into circulation in the cycle of matter, making nutrients available again for plants.

Mushrooms use 3 different evolutionary strategies to live. Depending on the nutritional needs, fungi are divided into saprophytes, symbionts and parasites.

Saprophytic fungi are those fungi that use animal and vegetable organic matter to grow and reproduce. Given their strategy, saprophytic mushrooms are the easiest to grow.

In fact, thanks to their enzymes, they are able to break down organic substances such as wood into assimilable substances for their growth. Given the high variability of fungi, there are many species capable of breaking down any organic substance in nature.

Symbiont fungi are those fungi that require the presence of a specific symbiont organism to survive. Symbiont fungi create a mutually beneficial bond with the host plant, initiating a continuous exchange of substances between fungus and host.

The most famous case of symbiotic mushroom is the porcini mushroom, the most sought after and valuable mushroom from a commercial point of view.

The cultivation of the porcini mushroom deserves a dedicated chapter, its cultivation is still in an experimental phase because the boletus, being a symbiotic fungus, needs the host plant appropriately mycorrhized.

The procedure is similar to the cultivation of truffles.

If you have entrepreneurial intentions, the cultivation of porcini is not the most suitable given the difficulty. To get started, you will need to devote yourself to the cultivation of saprophytic mushrooms.

If you want to learn more about the cultivation of symbiotic mushrooms, read the chapter: how to grow truffles.

The third group, that of parasites, are fungi that live and grow at the expense of other living organisms. In addition to nutritional strategies, mushrooms can be divided into microscopic and macroscopic, pathogenic and non-pathogenic, poisonous and edible fungi.

Fungi produce a myriad of chemical compounds that are used by humans in many sectors, from food to pharmaceuticals. The most famous case of use of mushrooms is that of Saccharomyces cerevisiae, or better known as brewer's yeast. Man can eat only a very small part of the mushrooms found in nature, and even fewer are the mushrooms cultivable by man.

Most of the mushrooms eaten by humans are collected in nature during the ripening period. In fact, the mushroom lives most of its life as a mycelium, and then generates the fruit, that is the mushroom as we know and use it.

Given the immense biodiversity, it is possible to find mushrooms in almost any environment and the collection is strictly regulated by the authorities because it is very easy to exchange an edible species for a poisonous one. There are several deadly species that can easily be mistaken for species suitable for consumption.

Mushroom picking is very popular because some of the most prized species (such as the porcini) are found only in nature and cannot be grown.

Edible mushrooms are widely used by the food industry, and for this reason mushroom cultivation has been developed and refined to meet the sustained market demand.

How to Grow Mushrooms. We have already seen that only some mushrooms are edible for humans, much less cultivable ones.

Furthermore, we have highlighted that among the various categories of mushrooms, the saprophytic ones are the most suitable for cultivation. There are many variables to consider when choosing which mushroom to market. If on the one hand the technical aspect is important, on the other hand it is essential to guarantee the profitability of the plant. Several species of mushrooms are cultivated all over the world, from Asia to America, but in Italy the cultivated species are few.

The most abundant and frequent species is undoubtedly the classic champignon mushroom (agaricus bisporus), followed by the oyster mushroom (Pleurotus ostreatus) and the poplar or poplar (Agrocybe aegerita).

All three fungi are obviously saprophytic, i.e. they grow using organic matter present in the substrate.

How to grow mushrooms

Mushroom farming can be carried out by anyone, from the citizen who wants to produce mushrooms at home for his own consumption, to the small agricultural entrepreneur looking for an additional source of income, and then to the large farm that invests millions in the construction of plant suitable for cultivation.

Depending on the type of investment, production can vary from a few specimens to tons of mushrooms per day. Whatever the quantity produced; mushrooms are grown following almost the same guidelines.

To grow properly, a mushroom needs the following characteristics:

- an appropriate substrate;
- the right degree of humidity and Ph;
- controlled temperature.

Given the difficulty of cultivating symbiotic mushrooms (Porcini), almost all of the plants are dedicated to saprophytic mushrooms. This type of fungi needs a suitable substrate where to enter the spores of the fungi.

Mushroom production is divided into two major stages: preparation of the substrate and growth of the fungus. The companies that carry out both operations operate closed-cycle cultivation, that is, they carry out all the operational phases of mushroom cultivation.

Closed loop companies are large companies because preparing the right substrate involves a significant investment in automatic machines and personnel. This situation has led some companies to specialize in the production of substrate to be sold to small businesses.

Depending on the species of mushroom grown, the substrate will vary in chemical and physical composition. Since the champignon mushroom is the most cultivated mushroom, I report the stages of its production. In general, however, the stages are similar in all cultivable saprophytic species.

Generally, abundant raw materials such as various types of manure, straw, hay, agricultural chalk and water are used to prepare the substrate.

This mixture of substances is suitably fermented in large machines until the complete maturation of the substrate, ready for the next step of pasteurization. This phase is necessary to eliminate competing mushrooms.

Once ready, the substrate is sown with the mycelium of the mushroom, divided into special packages and marketed to growers. By doing this, the small farmer can grow his own mushrooms while reducing start-up costs.

With the substrate ready, mushroom cultivation is relatively simple because it proceeds by itself, as long as the environmental conditions are respected.

After the arrival of the pallets of mycorrhized substrate, the grower must leave the compost at 25 ° for two weeks to allow the mycelium to grow inside the substrate. During this period, you will notice a change in the substrate, with the formation of a whitish layer. At this point, the mycelium has passed the incubation phase.

The substrate is covered with a special soil and left to mature for a further 10 days.

During these first 25 days, you will notice constant changes in the substrate in terms of smell and color. At this point, the time will come to pass from the vegetative to the reproductive phase, that is the birth of the fruit of the mushroom, the edible part.

To make the switch, you need to ventilate the room and lower the temperature to 16-18 °. After about a week you will see the first white tips of the fungus appear which in a couple of days will reach commercial size.

All these procedures are carried out inside specific cultivation greenhouses. These greenhouses are made with different materials and have automatic systems to control the climatic conditions. These structures are made so that the mushrooms are placed on different shelves to optimize the space. The total size of the greenhouse is variable, the important thing is to keep the temperature and humidity constant.

An agricultural entrepreneur who intends to cultivate only mushrooms must plan the construction of about 10 greenhouses of 100-200 square meters.

The figures are completely approximate, every good entrepreneur must predict the productivity of the plant in the start-up phase also thanks to the advice of expert growers.

HOW TO START A SUCCESSFUL MUSHROOM GROWING PLANT

Inventing a job, opening a business and becoming independent is one of the most beautiful and rewarding things we can do in life.

However, despite the apparent ease, setting up a business is difficult and entrepreneurs do not improvise. Before creating any project, you have to study a lot and invest in training.

Once the basic knowledge has been achieved, the concepts must be put into practice but with an approach that limits the initial investments.

A successful entrepreneur must know how to manage their emotions and start small. The road to success is made up of small and constant daily actions, not of rash steps disproportionate to one's abilities.

If you want to grow mushrooms professionally, reduce the entrepreneurial risk and start with a single greenhouse, this way you will take control of the technical operations without risking too much money.

Starting a small mushroom farm is ideal for all those farms looking for an alternative source of income and to attract customers to their business.

This practice is also very interesting for farms looking for visibility. You can offer training days to your guests in order to differentiate yourself from the competition.

In order to survive on the market, agricultural entrepreneurial activities must also appeal to final customers and the mushroom is very suitable for this type of approach.

Mushroom farming is a niche crop and people are increasingly interested in this type of business. Organize educational days, they will be an excellent promotional strategy.

Growing mushrooms: final thoughts

We have seen that mushroom growing is a very interesting agricultural activity, especially if we consider the relative ease and good profitability of the plants. For the moment the cultivable mushroom species are limited, however I am sure that in the coming years we will see an exponential growth of species suitable for cultivation. Technologies improve and also the interest of ordinary people in local, organic production. This sector is the future of human nutrition and I am sure that more and more people will turn to the local zero km market.

www.ingramcontent.com/pod-product-compliance
Lightning Source LLC
Chambersburg PA
CBHW060336030426
42336CB00011B/1377